Allergic Disease - New Developments in Diagnosis and Therapy

Edited by Öner Özdemir

Published in London, United Kingdom

Allergic Disease - New Developments in Diagnosis and Therapy
http://dx.doi.org/10.5772/intechopen.102204
Edited by Öner Özdemir

Contributors
Olga Lima Tavares Machado, Mariana Giarola Benedito Bartholazzi, Tatiana de Morais Lodi, Leisheng Zhang, Xiaowei Gao, Zhongchao Han, Franziska Zemmer, Fatih Ozkaragoz, Natalia Koshkarova, Natalia Cherevko, Andrew Klimov, Vladimir Klimov, Natalia Esakova, Alexander Nikolaevich Pampura, Venera Baybekova, Nazifa Dustbabaeva, Öner Özdemir, Emine Aylin Yilmaz, Maria C. Jimenez-Martínez, Henry Velazquez-Soto

First published in London, United Kingdom, 2023 by IntechOpen
IntechOpen is the global imprint of INTECHOPEN LIMITED, registered in England and Wales, registration number: 11086078, 5 Princes Gate Court, London, SW7 2QJ, United Kingdom

British Library Cataloguing-in-Publication Data
A catalogue record for this book is available from the British Library

Additional hard and PDF copies can be obtained from orders@intechopen.com

Allergic Disease - New Developments in Diagnosis and Therapy
Edited by Öner Özdemir
p. cm.
Print ISBN 978-1-80356-845-4
Online ISBN 978-1-80356-846-1
eBook (PDF) ISBN 978-1-80356-847-8

Meet the editor

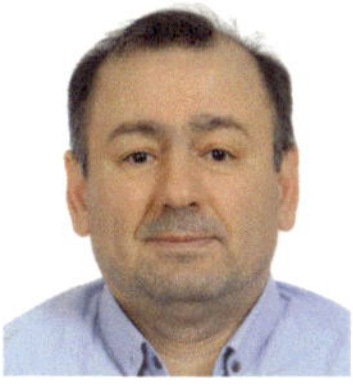

Prof. Dr. Öner Özdemir graduated with an MD degree from İstanbul Medical School, İstanbul University in 1989. He completed his pediatric residency at the Department of Pediatrics, Children's Hospital, İstanbul Medical School. He completed his clinical fellowship training in the Pediatric Allergy/Immunology division, at Louisiana State University, Health Sciences Centre, USA, and at the Pediatric Allergy/Immunology program, at Cincinnati Children's Hospital Medical Center, USA. Dr. Özdemir was the first-place winner of the 2005 Clemens Von Pirquet Award from the American College of Allergy, Asthma and Immunology (ACAAI) for the best research on allergy/asthma/immunology by a fellow in training. He has more than 250 international and national publications, 230 international and 180 national presentations, and more than 20 book chapters to his credit. He has also edited seven books.

Contents

Preface

This book includes eight chapters organized into four sections.

Chapter 1 introduces the topic. Chapter 2 discusses the basics of molecular allergy and the importance of a molecular biological approach in clinical allergy, especially in food and pollen allergies. Chapter 3 reviews the aerobiological approach and the contribution of aerobiology in the diagnosis and treatment of pollen allergy. Chapter 4 discusses food allergies, including cow's milk and egg food allergies. It also highlights new therapeutic methods for treating allergies (e.g., oral-sublingual route immunotherapy modalities) and preventive methods such as early administration of some foods. Chapter 5 is about anaphylaxis, which is one of the most serious complications of food allergies. The diagnostic description of anaphylaxis is always debatable and diagnosing anaphylaxis is challenging, especially in infants. Chapter 6 discusses allergen-specific immunotherapy, in which different therapeutic modalities (oral, sublingual, epidermal, intralymphatic, etc.) as well as different commercial preparations have been developed, especially for food and pollen allergies. Chapter 7 examines the novel treatment approach of mesenchymal stem/stromal cells, which is being tested for allergic diseases such as atopic dermatitis and chronic urticaria. Finally, Chapter 8 discusses the management of various allergic diseases during the COVID-19 pandemic.

I would like to thank the staff at IntechOpen, especially Author Service Managers Jasna Bozic and Dominik Samardzija for their assistance throughout the publication process.

Öner Özdemir, MD
Research and Training Hospital,
Division of Pediatric Allergy / Immunology,
Sakarya University Medical Faculty,
Sakarya, Türkiye

Section 1

Introductory

Chapter 1

Introductory Chapter: Allergic Disease – New Developments in Diagnosis and Therapy

Öner Özdemir

1. Introduction

In today's world of the allergy epidemic, this book will discuss primarily the changes and developments in the diagnosis and treatment of well-known allergic diseases in light of recent literature. Today, with the developing of technology, diagnosing allergic diseases is much more than just skin-prick tests and specific IgE examinations. Many things now require diagnosis at the molecular level and more appropriate diagnosis and proper treatments [1, 2].

2. Aim

In our book and in this brief section, we gave priority to the topics, which we encounter very often in the allergy outpatient clinic and the current developments in this field.

3. New developments in diagnosis and therapy of allergic diseases

Nowadays, the basic knowledge of molecular allergy is increasing very rapidly. The molecular biological approach is most useful today in the study of food allergies and cross-reactive allergens [3–5]. In light of the innovations in the literature on molecular allergy, the reflection of this from laboratory tests to bedside clinical practices is becoming more important every day.

Also, an aerobiological approach and the contribution of aerobiology in the diagnosis and treatment of pollen allergy are one of the developing areas. An aerobiological approach will not only give a more accurate diagnosis but will also help detect and treat more accurately the actual pollen to which the person may be allergic [6].

Food allergies, which are increasing day by day, are like a new challenge to our civilization. While we were talking about food allergies that disappeared at an earlier age and were not so stubborn and difficult to treat until recently, we can talk about food allergies that are more resistant to treatment, disappear at a later age, and generally it appears as multiple food allergies [7, 8]. In the past, cow's milk and egg food allergies were the most common and well-known types of food allergies that were relatively easy to treat. Again, apart from diet therapy, immunotherapy modalities that are tried by oral-sublingual route against various foods are very popular today. To reduce the frequency of food allergy development, early administration of some foods has also come to the fore today [9].

Again, the frequency of anaphylaxis, which is one of the serious problems in food allergies, and the chance of it appearing in the clinic is like the increase in the incidence of all other allergic diseases. Recently, there have been some changes in the definition of anaphylaxis, the diagnosis of which has always been controversial. Apart from hypotension, after exposure to certain/known allergens, the appearance of respiratory symptoms (e.g., laryngomalacia, and bronchospasm) was also accepted as anaphylaxis [10, 11]. Apart from the difficulties in diagnosing anaphylaxis, infant anaphylaxis is a difficult issue in its own right. As it is so difficult to evaluate and decide on anaphylaxis-related symptoms and signs in infants [12, 13], there has been no recent change in this treatment.

It is known that all allergic diseases occur through immune mediation. Again, although allergic diseases generally have a common immunopathogenesis, there may be minor variations specific to the individual disease. Allergen-specific immunotherapy is one of the most developed topics in allergy recently. Apart from the use of molecular allergy and aerobiological methods when planning immunotherapy [4], different methods have been developed as I mentioned above when talking about food allergy. In addition, application with other methods (oral, sublingual, epidermal, intralymphatic, etc.,) other than the classical method, the subcutaneous route, is partially becoming common in food as well as pollen allergies. Again, apart from orally administered liquid preparations, tablet-like and home allergen-specific immunotherapy applications are becoming widespread, especially for pollen and dust mite allergies [14, 15]. Various companies have preparations for this purpose, especially in European Union countries.

Besides allergen-specific immunotherapy, the use of mesenchymal stem/stromal cells is available today as trial treatments in many autoimmune, chronic diseases, even in COVID-19 other than allergic diseases. It has been first tried in mice, especially in atopic dermatitis, and its success has been reported [16]. It is very new to be tested for allergic diseases such as atopic dermatitis and chronic urticaria. Although this form of treatment looks promising, trials are new, and the chances of success are still low. But if it is successful, it may appear more frequently in the future as a radical and preventive treatment option [17].

4. Conclusion

I hope that the issues described in the light of the current information in this book will change the diagnostic and therapeutic approaches of allergists and lead to better and more accurate results for the patient.

I would be very glad that our book will be useful to all our readers...

Author details

Öner Özdemir
Research and Training Hospital of Sakarya University Faculty of Medicine, Division of Allergy and Immunology, Sakarya, Türkiye

*Address all correspondence to: ozdemir_oner@hotmail.com

References

[1] Strachan DP. Hay fever, hygiene, and household size. BMJ. 1989;**299**:1259-1260

[2] Bae JM. Interpretation of the hygiene and microflora hypothesis for allergic diseases through epigenetic epidemiology. Epidemiological Health. 2018;**40**:e2018006. DOI: 10.4178/epih.e2018006

[3] Volpicella M, Leoni C, Dileo MCG, Ceci LR. Progress in the analysis of food allergens through molecular biology approaches. Cell. 2019;**8**(9):1073. DOI: 10.3390/cells8091073

[4] Izmailovich M, Semenova Y, Abdushukurova G, Mukhamejanova A, Dyussupova A, Faizova R, et al. Molecular aspects of allergen-specific immunotherapy in patients with seasonal allergic rhinitis. Cell. 2023;**12**(3):383. DOI: 10.3390/cells12030383

[5] Huang Z, Zou X, Chen H, Liao C, Hu H, Luo W, et al. Identifying potential co-sensitization and cross-reactivity patterns based on component-resolved diagnosis. International Archives of Allergy and Immunology. 2020;**181**(2):81-93. DOI: 10.1159/000504320

[6] Markey E, Clancy JH, Martínez-Bracero M, Maya-Manzano JM, Smith M, Skjøth C, et al. A comprehensive aerobiological study of the airborne pollen in the Irish environment. Aerobiologia (Bologna). 2022;**38**(3):343-366. DOI: 10.1007/s10453-022-09751-w

[7] Anvari S, Miller J, Yeh CY, Davis CM. IgE-mediated food allergy. Clinical Reviews in Allergy and Immunology. 2019;**57**(2):244-260. DOI: 10.1007/s12016-018-8710-3

[8] Valenta R, Hochwallner H, Linhart B, Pahr S. Food allergies: The basics. Gastroenterology. 2015;**148**(6):1120. DOI: 10.1053/j.gastro.2015.02.006

[9] Nuyttens L, De Vlieger L, Diels M, Schrijvers R, Bullens DMA. The clinical and immunological basis of early food introduction in food allergy prevention. Frontiers in Allergy. 2023;**4**:1111687. DOI: 10.3389/falgy.2023.1111687

[10] Cardona V, Ansotegui IJ, Ebisawa M, El-Gamal Y, Fernandez Rivas M, Fineman S, et al. World allergy organization anaphylaxis guidance 2020. World Allergy Organization Journal. 2020;**13**(10):100472. DOI: 10.1016/j.waojou.2020.100472

[11] Tarczoń I, Cichocka-Jarosz E, Knapp A, Kwinta P. The 2020 update on anaphylaxis in pediatric population. Postepy Dermatological Aerology. 2022;**39**(1):13-19. DOI: 10.5114/ada.2021.103327

[12] Cardenas-Morales M, Hernandez-Trujillo V. Infant anaphylaxis: A diagnostic challenge. Current Allergy and Asthma Reports. 2021;**21**(2):12. DOI: 10.1007/s11882-021-00990-4

[13] Arıkoğlu T, Ozhan AK, Kuyucu S. Management of anaphylaxis in pediatric population. Current Pharmaceutical Design. 2023;**29**(3):209-223. DOI: 10.2174/1381612829666221021154032

[14] Nowak-Wegrzyn A, Sato S, Fiocchi A, Ebisawa M. Oral and sublingual immunotherapy for food allergy. Current Opinion in Allergy and Clinical Immunology. 2019;**19**(6):606-613. DOI: 10.1097/ACI.0000000000000587

[15] Meltzer EO, Wallace D, Friedman HS, Navaratnam P, Scott EP, Nolte H. Meta-analyses of the efficacy of pharmacotherapies and sublingual allergy immunotherapy tablets for allergic rhinitis in adults and children. Rhinology. 2021;**59**(5):422-432. DOI: 10.4193/Rhin21.054

[16] Lee BC, Kim JJ, Lee JY, Kang I, Shin N, Lee SE, et al. Disease-specific primed human adult stem cells effectively ameliorate experimental atopic dermatitis in mice. Theranostics. 2019;**9**(12):3608-3621. DOI: 10.7150/thno.32945

[17] Kim EY, Kim HS, Hong KS, Chung HM, Park SP, Noh G. Mesenchymal stem/stromal cell therapy in atopic dermatitis and chronic urticaria: Immunological and clinical viewpoints. Stem Cell Research & Therapy. 2021;**12**(1):539. DOI: 10.1186/s13287-021-02583-4

Section 2

Allergy Essentials

Chapter 2

Fundamentals of Molecular Allergy: From Bench to Bedside

Henry Velázquez-Soto and Maria C. Jimenez Martinez

Abstract

This chapter describes the fundamentals of molecular allergy diagnosis and raises the concept of allergens, allergenic components, and recombinant allergens. In addition, the authors review quality aspects related to the laboratory methodology. In the last part of the chapter, the different singleplex and multiplex platforms currently used for molecular diagnosis are compared. Finally, the diagnostic systems' challenges, strengths, and pitfalls are discussed to understand their clinical impact. Undoubtedly, this chapter will be handy for the background knowledge for health personnel, allergists/immunologists, and clinical laboratory personnel to guide the selection of diagnostic tests for allergy as well as their interpretation and therapeutic approach.

Keywords: molecular allergy, laboratory tests, allergens, allergy diagnostic

1. Introduction

Allergies are one of the most prevalent diseases affecting almost one billion people worldwide [1]. The traditional approaches for identifying allergen-specific IgE have undergone a revolution as a result of the growing need for the best diagnostic techniques, technological advancements, and understanding of allergen structure and obtention. These technical and scientific advances are the fundamentals of molecular diagnosis and precision medicine in allergy [2, 3].

2. Principles of laboratory testing for molecular allergy

Immunoglobulin E (IgE) is one of the five immunoglobulin isotypes described in humans and is considered to mediate hypersensitivity type I reactions and be the main soluble molecule involved in allergy pathology [4]. This immunoglobulin has historically been recognized as a biomarker for allergic processes. Due to its feasibility to detect and measure in serum samples, several laboratory methods focus on the identification of total IgE (tIgE), and specific IgE (sIgE) [5].

Measurements of tIgE and sIgE are based on antigen-antibody reactions. For tIgE detection, an anti-IgE antibody (detection antibody) will bind to the fragment crystallizable region in the immunoglobulin E. For sIgE, the serum sample is incubated with the allergen-coated surface before incubation with the detection antibody, thus allowing allergen-specific IgE to be detected. Finally, the reaction is detected according to the platform methodology: radiation, colorimetry, fluorometry, or chemiluminescence [6–8].

2.1 Units and equivalences

Serum IgE is usually found in very low concentrations ranging <1μg/mL. Most immunoassay systems now use a total calibration curve that is associated with the World Health Organization (WHO) IgE standard and reported in arbitrary units; for better comprehension, tIgE is reported in IU/ml or kIU/L, which is equivalent to 2.4 ng/ml; [9] while sIgE is reported in kUA/L (kUA/L kilo mass units of allergenspecific antibody per unit volume) [10].

2.2 Methodologies for tIgE and sIgE determination

The evolution of methods for IgE diagnostic comprises methods like Radio-Immuno-Sorbent-Test (RAST), Paper-Radio-Immuno-Sorbent-Test (PRIST), and Enzyme-Linked Immuno-Sorbent-Assay (ELISA), gave rise to more reliable, safe, and automatized methods. A deeper revision of these methodologies could be found in [6].

2.3 Current methodologies used for sIgE determination

2.3.1 Enzyme-linked-immuno-sorbent assay (ELISA)

ELISA protocols are based on colorimetric reactions. Allergen is bound to the plate, then the sample of the patient containing IgE is incubated, allowing it to react with the allergen, forming the first antigen-antibody complex. Then a secondary antibody linked to an oxidizing enzyme binds to the previously formed complex, and by addition of the substrate, the color begins to develop. Finally, the plate is read in a spectrophotometer to detect the absorbance, which is proportional to the sIgE concentration (**Figure 1**) [11].

2.3.2 Immunoblot

For immunoblot-based methods, antigens are bound to a polymeric membrane acting as the solid phase, allowing IgE to interact with the different allergens. Then a phosphatase alkaline-linked secondary antibody is added to the reaction. Finally, the substrate precipitates leaving colored marks in the spots where patient´s IgE reacted with allergen (**Figure 1**) [12].

2.3.3 Chemiluminescence

The method for chemiluminescence platforms is very similar to ELISA. Alkaline phosphatase, which is linked to the secondary antibody, produces chemiluminescence signals when it reacts with its substrate, the phosphate ester of adamantyl dioxetane. In this method, the intensity of chemiluminescence is proportional to sIgE concentration (**Figure 1**) [13].

DOI: http://dx.doi.org/10.5772/intechopen.107512

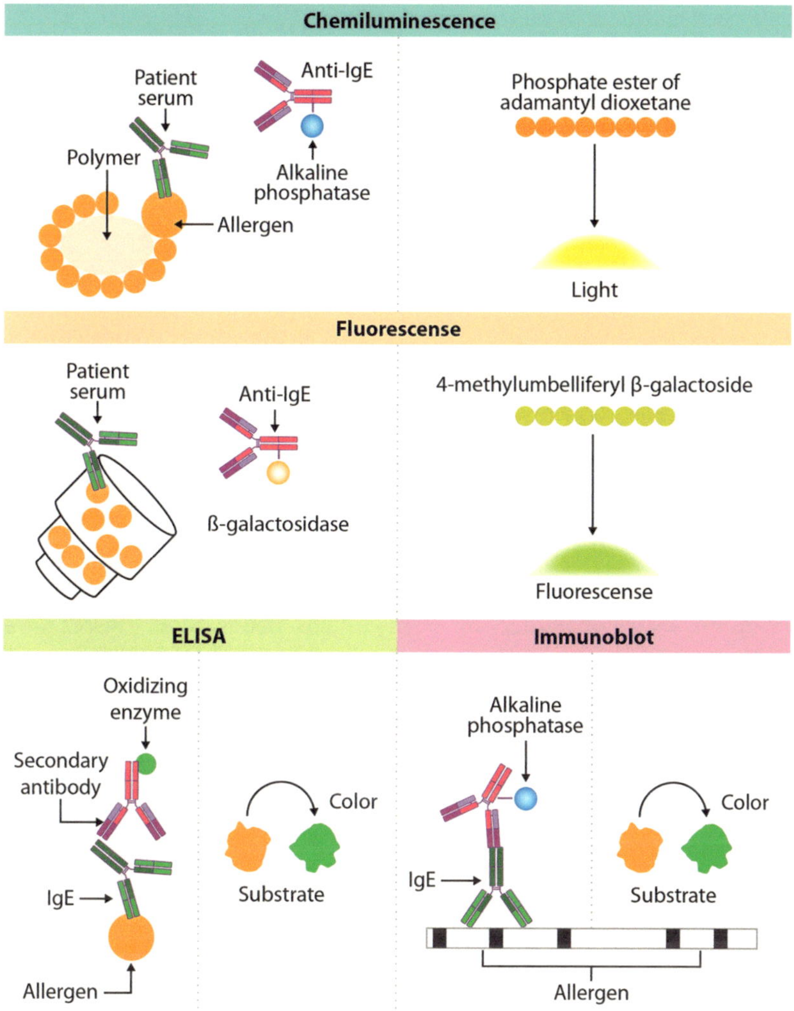

Figure 1.
Fundamentals of current methods for IgE detection. Different techniques are used to determine tIgE and sIgE in patients' samples; all of them are based on Ag-Ab reaction.

2.3.4 Fluoro-enzyme-immunoassay (FEIA)

In FEIA techniques, the secondary antibody is coupled to galactosidase, which reacts with 4-methylumbelliferyl βgalactoside to generate fluorescence proportional to the amount of specific IgE in the sample (**Figure 1**) [14].

3. Singleplex platforms for IgE determinations

Singleplex platforms permit the determination and quantification of tIgE or sIgE. In the case of sIgE determinations, these instruments identify one allergen per reaction.

Singleplex devices usually include the following components: [2, 14]

1. An allergen platform in solid or liquid phase.

2. A reaction container in which human serum or controls are exposed to anti-IgE detection reagent.

3. Calibration, data acquisition, processing, and analysis systems.

3.1 ImmunoCAP Phadia by ThermoFisher

It was the first automated platform using FEIA as the operating principle, showing high concordance with RAST in its results. Phadia 250 has a processing capacity of 60 tests per hour and allows the use of native and recombinant allergenic components which are grouped within the ImmunoCAP line, such as grass pollens, weed pollens, tree pollens, microorganisms, animal proteins, and mites, among others [15, 16].

3.2 Immulite by Siemens

Immulite is an IgE detection platform based on chemiluminescence. This equipment determines a variety of allergens from animals, drugs, food, grasses, insects, mites, mold, parasites, trees, and weeds, among others. It also includes a panel of 26 recombinant allergenic components. Immulite 2000 is capable of processing up to 200 results per hour and with a sensitivity of up to 0.1 kU/L [17, 18].

3.3 Hytec 288 by Hycor Biomedical

Hytec 288 is an immunoassay instrument based on ELISA. This platform offers the determination of single allergens and allergen mixture from drugs, food, grasses/weeds, animal proteins, among others. This equipment could perform up to 288 tests per run [19].

These three platforms are the leaders in the global market and exhibit excellent analytic sensitivity, precision, reproducibility, and linearity in total and allergen-specific IgE assays, but some variability in allergen-specific IgE quantitative estimates [16, 19].

4. Multiplex platforms for IgE determinations

Multiplex immunoassays allow for the identification of IgE sensitization repertoires against a diverse set of allergens. In contrast to singleplex platforms, the results are semiquantitative and not interchangeable. Characteristics of both platforms can be seen in **Table 1.**

4.1 Immuno solid-phase allergen chip (ISAC), by Thermo Fisher

The immuno solid-phase allergen chip (ImmunoCAP-ISAC) was the first multiplex platform designed and approved for IgE identification. This platform is based on the FEIA on-chip methodology, which can identify up to 112 allergenic components from 48 different allergen sources in approximately 4 hours. The ISAC system employs ISAC standardized units (ISU-E) ranging from 0.3 to 100 ISU-E, equivalent

	Singleplex	Multiplex
Results	**Quantitative**	**Semi quantitative**
Allergens tested per run	Depends on platform	Up to 178
Test result time	60 per hour- 200 per hour for individual tests	4h for whole panels
Cost	Cheap (if testing for few allergens)	Expensive
Personnel	Laboratory Technician	High-trained Laboratory Technician

Table 1.
Comparison between singleplex and multiplex platforms.

to 0.3–100 kUa/L, to categorize sIgE concentration into four groups: undetectable or very low (0.3 kUA/L), low (0.3 to 13 kUA/L), moderate to high (13 to 153 kUA/L), and very high (153 kUA/L) (**Figure 2**) [11, 20].

4.2 EUROLINE by Euroimmune

Euroline is a semiquantitative based immunoblot instrument. It provides pre-coated membranes for detecting sIgE from various allergen sources. These precoated membrane panels are tailored to the clinically relevant allergens in the regions where these are commercialized. Interestingly, this platform offers reagents for diminishing cross-reactive carbohydrate determinants (CCD), improving sensitivity. The number of allergens detectable in one membrane varies depending on the panel in use (8–45 allergens). The results can be obtained in a lapse of approximately two hours [21].

4.3 Allergy Explorer (ALEX) by Macro Array Diagnostics

The Allergy Explorer platform was the first to use an ELISA-based methodology to determine tIgE and sIgE levels for 117 extracts and 178 recombinant allergens at

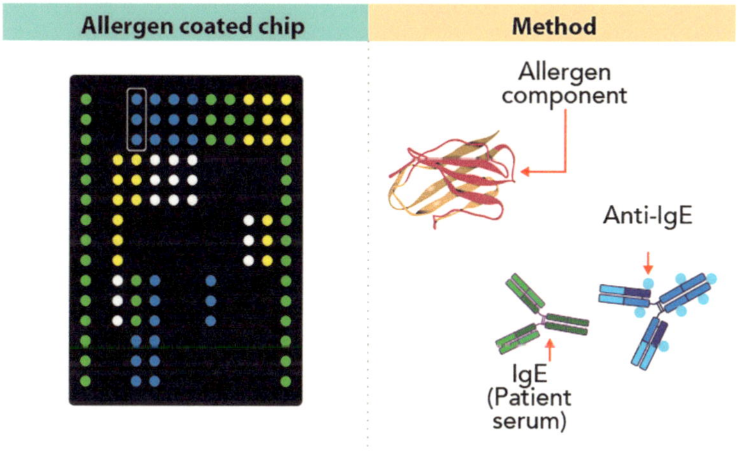

Figure 2.
Immuno solid-phase allergen chip (ISAC). Multiplex immunoassay based on FEIA methodology.

the same time. This device can block the determination of clinically irrelevant sIgE directed against CCD. The platform has manual and automated processing formats, with the capacity to analyze up to 50 patients in an approximate time of 4 hours. ALEX contains pre-designed panels by a group of symptoms or group of allergens, such as grass pollens, dander allergens, epithelium of animals, mites and cockroaches, molds, and yeasts.

The results of the tests are presented graphically, including the allergen's name, the specific allergen component or extract, the biological function, and the reported sIgE concentration in kUA/L. The final report includes a demonstration of possible cross-sensitization as well as interpretation and medical follow-up recommendations for the treating physician. ALEX employs a classification based on the concentration of sIgE obtained: Negative or uncertain (0.3 kUA/L), low (0.3 to 1 kUA/L), moderate (1–5 kUA/L), high (5–15 kUA/L), and very high (> 15 kUA/L) (See **Figure 3**) [22].

These three instruments evaluate the eight most common allergen families: Bet v 1-related protein (PR-10); Venom group 5 allergen family; Cupin Superfamily; EF-hand domain (Ca++ binding proteins); Expansin C-terminal domain; Lipocalin; Profilin; and Prolamin superfamily [20–22].

Although evaluated in different allergic diseases with patients sensitized to different allergens its performance, sensitivity and specificity have been reviewed and tested by different authors (**Table 2**) [8, 23, 24].

5. Allergens, allergenic extracts, and allergen components.

As mentioned above, laboratory diagnosis relies on antigen-antibody reactions, with the allergen defining the IgE specificity. Therefore, it is essential to emphasize the concepts of allergen, source, and obtention methods.

5.1 Allergens

Allergens are any molecule that binds to IgE antibodies [25]. Allergens are immunogenic antigens that induce a robust Th2 response, characterized by high IL-4 and IL-13 production with secretion of IgE [26].

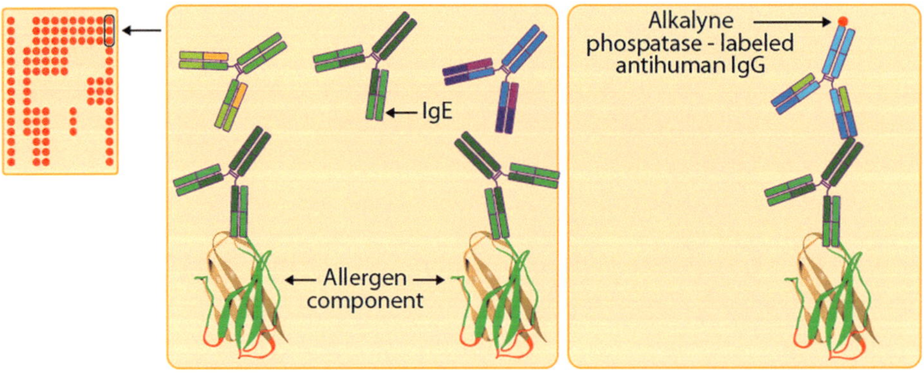

Figure 3.
Allergy Explorer (ALEX). Multiplex immunoassay based on ELISA technique.

	ALEX	ISAC	EUROLINE
Allergens or components tested per run	117–178	112	Up to 45
Test result time	4 h	4 h	3h (time optimized), 3.5 h (time/volume optimized), 14–26 h (volume/time optimized)
Sensitivity	93%*	86%**	31–88.9%***
Specificity	100%*	100%**	70–96.7%***
Methodology	ELISA	Fluorescence	Blot

**Evaluated in tree nut allergy.*
***Systematic review.*
****Compared to skin prick test.*

Table 2.
Comparison of multiplex platforms.

5.2 Allergen extracts

Allergen extracts (AEs) are complex mixtures of allergenic and nonallergenic molecules, including proteins, lipids, saccharides, nucleic acids, lipids, low molecular weight metabolites, pigments, and salts. AEs are obtained from natural sources such as pollens, animals, and insects, using physical methods (grinding) or chemical methods (solvents). Based on their intended application, allergen extracts should be characterized and subjected to quality control. As a result, validated assays must be developed to ensure the presence of relevant allergens for diagnostic or therapeutic applications (**Figure 4**) [27, 28].

5.3 Allergen components

Allergen components are isolated proteins derived from a purified extract of a specific allergenic source. These allergens, whether native or recombinant, are generally homogeneous and subject to stringent quality control [14].

Recombinant allergens are the most effective approach for obtaining allergen components. These highly pure allergens are produced by biotechnology; the process begins with cDNA obtention from mRNA through reverse transcription. Then, the cDNA may be modified (point mutations, chimeras/hybrids, fragmentation, oligomerization) to obtain the most accurate allergen molecule. Subsequently, the cDNA is inserted into expression vectors, usually *E. coli*. or *P. pastoris*, to express the protein and obtain the recombinant allergen. The allergen is then isolated, purified, evaluated, and validated for its usage in diagnostic platforms or to be used as a hypoallergenic allergens for immunotherapy (**Figure 5**) [29].

5.4 Structural importance of allergens

5.4.1 Proteins

Proteins constitute the vast majority of allergens, but only a few allergens bind IgE antibodies in the serum of most allergic patients. These molecules are known as “major allergens.” A major allergen is defined as an antigen that binds to IgE in 50%

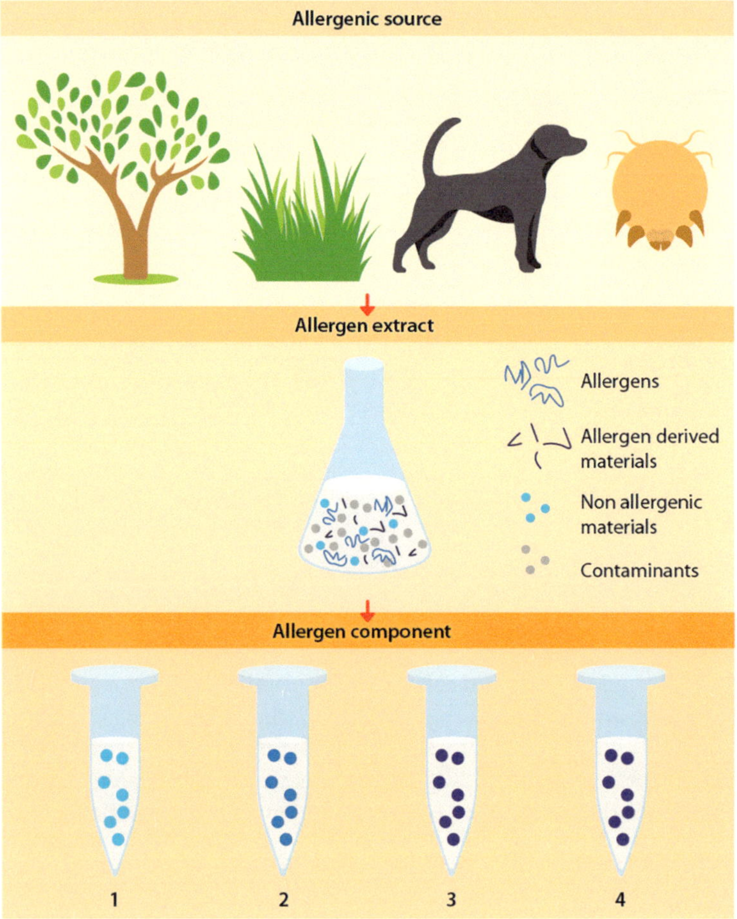

Figure 4.
Obtention of allergen extracts and allergen components from allergenic sources. Different techniques are used to obtain allergen extracts from diverse allergen sources. Most allergen extracts contain sensitizing allergen, allergen-derived materials, non-allergenic components, and contaminants. Following the obtention of allergen extracts, allergen components are isolated and purified, and protein characterization is performed.

or more of clinically allergic patients' serum. Other antigens that account for less than half of IgE binding are known as "minor allergens." Identifying major allergens has aided in understanding the immune response during allergic reactions, sensitization in atopy, and diagnostic applications.

5.4.2 Carbohydrates

Specific IgE antibodies for oligosaccharides are present in some patients, these antibodies cause numerous cross-reactions in vitro, given the designation cross-reactive carbohydrate determinants (CCDs). However, in recent years, oligosaccharide epitopes have been implicated in allergic sensitization, acute allergic reactions, and not just cross-reactions; consequently, characterization and discovery of glycan allergens have been a challenge. Currently, there are about approximately 20 oligosaccharides found in pollens, venoms, nematodes, worms, and ticks that are distributed in five glycans groups and have been shown to be significant for allergic disease [30].

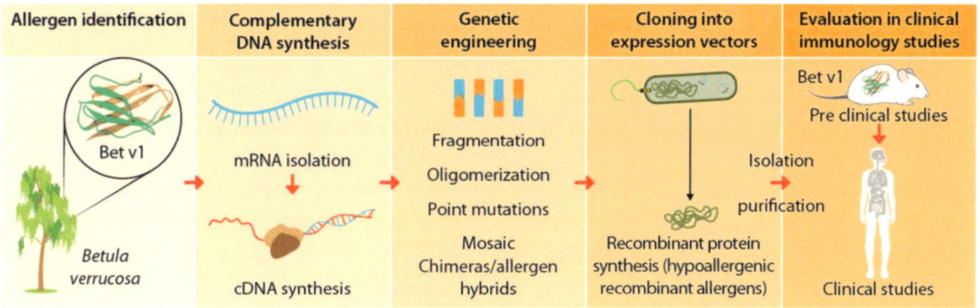

Figure 5.
Obtention of recombinant allergens. Recombinant allergens are obtained by isolating the mRNA from the allergenic source. Then transcribed into cDNA and inserted in bacteria or yeasts to allow its expression. Finally, clinical validation is needed to be used for diagnosis in vitro or in vivo.

5.4.3 Major groups

Group A. Cross-reactive carbohydrate determinants. Most CCDs are N-glycans, characterized by a basic structure of two GlcNAc with two or three terminal mannose residues. Allergens with these glycans are *Ole e* 1, *Api g* 5, *Bla g* 2 [30, 31].

Group B. Mammalian non-human oligosaccharides. The glycan structures described in this group are the disaccharide galactose-alpha-1,3-galactose, and the monosaccharide N-glycolyl neuraminic acid. These glycans are related to anaphylaxis and could be fond in red meat, tick bites, and some monoclonal antibodies [32, 33].

5.4.4 Minor groups

Group C. Oligosaccharides with O-linkage. O-glycans are oligosaccharides attached to serine or threonine residues on a protein and sometimes to tyrosine, hydroxylysine, or hydroxyproline. Examples of allergens expressing O-glycans are *Art v* 1, *Amb a* 4 [32].

Group D: Oligosaccharide Epitopes expressed on Schistosomes and other Helminths. These oligosaccharides have a single terminal galactose or N-acetylgalactosamine residue (GalNAc), keeping a molecular similarity to CCDs. Their clinical significance is still under study since alpha-1, 3-fucose epitope could be implicated with a paradoxical protective effect in asthmatic patients [34].

Group E. Short-chain galactooligosaccharides (GOS). GOS are usually produced by bacterial beta-galactosidase and occur naturally in milk processed with prebiotics. They are typically a chain of 2 to 6 galactose molecules attached to glucose and have been recognized in allergic reactions [30, 32].

5.4.5 Lipids

Lipid antigens are much less understood than carbohydrate antigens, they have been shown a direct effect on allergenic potential and cause allergic responses. For example, lipids delay the enzymatic digestion of Ara h 8 allowing this molecule to reach the intestinal immune system and favoring sensitization. Conversely, lipid-associated allergens such as Der p 2, Der p 5, and Der p 7 have been related to increased asthma symptoms and severe allergic reactions [35]. Thus, the application of sIgE determination against lipids is limited.

6. Interpretation, clinical applications, and limitations for molecular allergy

Even though the first cases of pollen-induced hay fever were documented in the early 1800s, it was not until 100 years later that a relationship to a serum factor called reagin was discovered (IgE) [4]. In the mid-1960s, allergy diagnosis was primarily relied on skin testing, and allergen extracts were far from standardized. However, developing recombinant allergens and starting allergen cloning between 1988 – 1995 created new opportunities for studying and diagnosing allergy disorders [29, 36, 37]. Molecular allergy is the practical application of these advances, allowing us to manage patients with high accuracy, and leading into the era of precision medicine.

6.1 Singleplex *vs.* multiplex immunoassays

As previously discussed, singleplex assays allow detection of IgE antibodies specific to the allergens identified in the patient's clinical history. A multiplex platform, in contrast, enables defining a person's IgE reaction to the whole range of allergens arrayed on a chip.

The main benefit of the singleplex immunoassays is that it measures the allergen-specific IgE antibody level in kilounits per liter (kUA/L) based on a total IgE calibration system that can be traced back to a human reference preparation from the WHO. The assay has high precision and reproducibility, reporting values as low as 0.1 kUA/L (range, 0.1–100 kUA/L), without interference of allergen-specific IgG antibodies.

Compared to multiplex immunoassays, singleplex assays have fewer allergen molecules available, give an incomplete IgE reactivity profile with just one or a few tests, are more expensive if more than one measurement needs to be taken, and need a larger amount of serum [38]. In contrast, multiplex assays are semiquantitative and provide a comprehensive IgE pattern using only a small volume of serum, which could be useful in the evaluation of polysensitized patients; but are only available in laboratories with high-end machinery with highly trained personnel, delaying results by days or weeks **(Table 3)** [39, 40].

Molecular immunoassays have some advantages over *in vivo* assays, such as the ability to be performed regardless of extensive skin disease or medications used, minor pain or anxiety- provoking in children, little patient cooperation required, and no risk to the patient. The fact that the whole allergen of a fresh allergen is more sensitive than purified allergen components is one of the limitations of molecular diagnosis compared to *in vivo* evaluation, this is particularly important if the goal is to perform allergen-specific immunotherapy [39, 40]. In contrast, advances in molecular allergy have enabled the development of vaccines based on recombinant DNA technology and synthetic peptide chemistry that could be monitored with sIgE or sIgG determinations throughout treatment [41].

6.2 Clinical allergy *vs.* sensitization

The majority of allergens, but not all, are sensitizing, which is defined as the capacity to induce allergen-specific IgE antibodies. Non-sensitizing allergens can only cause allergic symptoms if the individual has been sensitized to a cross-reactive allergen [3]. Cross-reactivity defines an antigen attribute intrinsically related to the allergen molecular characteristics that determine immune recognition by IgE.

	Singleplex immunoassays	Multiplex Immunoassays
Number of allergens	Limited, selected according to clinical history.	Complete profile of allergens, useful in polysensitized patients.
Preferred for cross- reactivity suspicion	No	Yes
Preferred for immunotherapy selection	No	Yes
Preferred for patients with well-known sensitization history	Yes	No
Cross-reactive carbohydrate determinants (CCDs) evaluation	No	Yes

Table 3.
Variables to consider when the molecular diagnosis is selected for the clinician: Singleplex vs. Multiplex instruments.

Identification of cross-reactivity is critical to detect patients with a high risk of anaphylaxis for example in peanut and tree nuts or seeds allergy. Other cases of cross-reactivity are latex and food, that is, banana, avocado, kiwi, and chestnut; and cross-reactivity between shellfish and insects due to chitins, specifically tropomyosin in dust mites

The precise point at which a sensitizing allergen causes clinical symptoms is determined by several factors such as quantity, exposure route, antigen structural characteristics, genetics, microbiota, innate or adaptative immune interactions, and microenvironment, among others. Thus, identifying an IgE-mediated mechanism is a critical step that directs avoidance measures and suitable pharmacological treatment. However, positive skin tests or specific IgE assay results do not always indicate that an allergen is causing symptoms; the clinical significance of allergen exposure and its relationship to symptoms must be established by examining the patient's medical history.

6.3 Allergen extracts *vs.* recombinant allergens

Although diagnostic assays based on purified recombinant allergens are becoming more popular, extracts from natural allergen sources continue to be widely used. The composition of an allergenic extract has a significant influence on the results of any IgE-based immunoassay.

Allergen extracts used in some platforms are made up of a variety of allergens, some of which have little or no clinical significance, such as carbohydrate epitopes in peanut or timothy grass pollen, which might result in false positive findings [38]. The use of allergenic extracts allows to precisely detect the specificity of the IgE in a patient's sample, but also permits the evaluation of only clinically relevant components from allergenic sources.

In the other hand, protein characterization of allergens has been fundamental to understand IgE cross-reactivity data in the absence of allergen-antibody complexes. Some of the benefits of recombinant allergens include increased diagnostic accuracy, the ability to distinguish genuine sensitization from cross-reactivity, the ability to evaluate the type and risk of an allergic reaction, and the ability to select patients and suitable allergens for immunotherapy [29, 42].

7. Conclusions

Personalized therapy based on genetic, immunologic, and functional endotyping, defined as the examination of a biological or pathological process, including therapeutic response through biomarkers determination, is part of the new treatment advances for allergy patients known as precision medicine. As previously discussed, a correct diagnosis is critical in these therapeutical approaches. In the case of molecular allergy, the choice of testing is influenced by several variables, including test accessibility, clinical history, technical constraints, type of allergen, immunoassay accuracy, single or multiplex platforms, and most importantly, the clinical question that the analysis pretends to resolve.

Finally, despite molecular diagnosis is an excellent tool for selecting the appropriate allergens for immunotherapy, minimizing potential test-related complications, evaluating polysensitization with difficult interpretation, and possibly predicting clinical outcomes. Unfortunately, the high cost, access limited in low-income countries, restricted availability due to regulatory affairs in others, and a lack of sufficient clinical studies with recombinant allergens keep molecular allergy out of reach for routine use, but with a promising future once these limitations are overcome.

Acknowledgements

Thanks to Jesús Mendoza for designing and drawing the chapter figures.

Funding

This work was partially supported by the Conde de Valenciana Foundation and the Department of Biochemistry, Faculty of Medicine, UNAM.

Conflict of interest

The authors declare no conflict of interest.

Fundamentals of Molecular Allergy: From Bench to Bedside
DOI: http://dx.doi.org/10.5772/intechopen.107512

Author details

Henry Velázquez-Soto[1] and Maria C. Jimenez Martinez[1,2]*

1 Department of Immunology and Research Unit, Institute of Ophthalmology "Conde de Valenciana Foundation", Mexico City, Mexico

2 Faculty of Medicine, Department of Biochemistry, National Autonomous University of Mexico, Mexico City, Mexico

*Address all correspondence to: mcjimenezm@facmed.unam.mx

References

[1] Agache I, Akdis CA. Precision medicine and phenotypes, endotypes, genotypes, regiotypes, and theratypes of allergic diseases. The Journal of Clinical Investigation. 2019;**129**(4):1493-1503

[2] Kleine-Tebbe J, Jappe U. Molecular allergy diagnostic tests: Development and relevance in clinical practice. Alsic. 2017;**1**(2):169-189

[3] Matricardi PM, Dramburg S, Potapova E, Skevaki C, Renz H. Molecular diagnosis for allergen immunotherapy. The Journal of Allergy and Clinical Immunology. 2019;**143**(3):831-843

[4] Ishizaka K, Ishizaka T. Identification of IgE. The Journal of Allergy and Clinical Immunology. 2016;**137**(6):1646-1650

[5] Platts-Mills TAE. The continuing effect of the discovery of IgE by Kimishige Ishizaka. The Journal of Allergy and Clinical Immunology. 2018;**142**(3):788-789

[6] Salazar A, Velázquez-Soto H, Ayala-Balboa J, Jiménez-Martínez MC. Allergen-based diagnostic: Novel and old methodologies with new approaches. In: Athari SS, editor. Allergen. London: InTech; 2017

[7] Wachholz PA, Dearman RJ, Kimber I. Detection of allergen-specific IgE antibody responses. Journal of Immunotoxicology. 2005;**1**(3-4):189-199

[8] Wongpiyabovorn J, Suratannon N, Boonmee S, Chatchatee P. Comparison of specific IgE detection by immunoblotting and fluorescence enzyme assay with in vivo skin prick test. Asian Pacific Journal of Allergy Immunology. 2018;**36**(3):159-165

[9] Seagroatt V, Anderson SG. The second international reference preparation for human serum immunoglobulin E and the first British standard for human serum immunoglobulin E. Journal of Biological Standardization. 1981;**9**(4):431-437

[10] Thorpe SJ, Heath A, Fox B, Patel D, Egner W. The 3rd International Standard for serum IgE: International collaborative study to evaluate a candidate preparation. Clinical Chemistry and Laboratory Medicine. 2014;**52**(9):93

[11] Alhajj M, Farhana A. Enzyme Linked Immunosorbent Assay. Treasure Island (FL): StatPearls Publishing; 2022

[12] Gallagher S, Chakavarti D. Immunoblot analysis. JoVE. 2008;**16**:759

[13] Cinquanta L, Fontana DE, Bizzaro N. Chemiluminescent immunoassay technology: What does it change in autoantibody detection? Autoimmune Highlights. 2017;**8**(1):9

[14] Popescu FD, Vieru M. Precision medicine allergy immunoassay methods for assessing immunoglobulin E sensitization to aeroallergen molecules. WJM. 2018;**8**(3):17-36

[15] Kelso JM, Sodhi N, Gosselin VA, Yunginger JW. Diagnostic performance characteristics of the standard Phadebas RAST, modified RAST, and pharmacia CAP system versus skin testing. Annals of Allergy. 1991;**67**(5):511-514

[16] Ansotegui IJ, Melioli G, Canonica GW, Caraballo L, Villa E, Ebisawa M, et al. IgE allergy diagnostics and other relevant tests in allergy, a World Allergy Organization position

paper. World Allergy Organization Journal. 2020;**13**(2):100080

[17] Siemens. IMMULITE 2000 XPi Immunoassay System. 2022

[18] Li TM, Chuang T, Tse S, Hovanec-Burns D, El Shami AS. Development and validation of a third generation allergen-specific IgE assay on the continuous random access. Annals of Clinical and Laboratory Science. 2000;**34**(1):67-74

[19] Hamilton RG. Proficiency survey-based evaluation of clinical total and allergen-specific IgE assay performance. Archives of Pathology & Laboratory Medicine. 2010;**134**(7):975-982

[20] Thermofisher Scientific. https://www.thermofisher.com/phadia/wo/en/our-solutions/immunocap-allergy-solutions/specific-ige-multiplex.html

[21] EUROINMUN AG. https://www.euroimmun.com/products/techniques/immunoblot/

[22] Macroarray Diagnostics: MADx. https://www.macroarraydx.com/products/alex

[23] Akarsu A, Ocak M, Sahiner UM, Soyer O, Sekerel BE. Multiplex component-based allergen macroarray test is useful to predict clinical reactivity to tree nuts in children. Allergology International. 2022;**71**(2):236-247

[24] Westwood M, Ramaekers B, Lang S, Armstrong N, Noake C, de Kock S, et al. ImmunoCAP® ISAC and Microtest for multiplex allergen testing in people with difficult to manage allergic disease: A systematic review and cost analysis. Health Technology Assessment. 2016;**20**(67):1-178

[25] Aalberse RC. Structural biology of allergens. The Journal of Allergy and Clinical Immunology. 2000;**106**(2):228-238

[26] Pavon L, Jiménez-Martinez MC, Garcés ME. Inmunologia Molecular, Celular y Traslacional. 2a ed. Wolters Kluwer Health; 2020

[27] Valenta R, Karaulov A, Niederberger V, Zhernov Y, Elisyutina O, Campana R, et al. Allergen extracts for in vivo diagnosis and treatment of allergy: Is there a future? The Journal of Allergy and Clinical Immunology: In Practice. 2018;**6**(6):1845-1855

[28] Faisal M, Vasiljevic T, Donkor ON. A review on methodologies for extraction, identification and quantification of allergenic proteins in prawns. Foodservice Research International. 2019;**121**:307-318

[29] Tscheppe A, Breiteneder H. Recombinant Allergens in Structural Biology, Diagnosis, and Immunotherapy. International Archives of Allergy and Immunology. 2017;**172**(4):187-202

[30] WHO/IUIS Allergen Nomenclature Sub-Committee. Glycan Epitopes Currently Recognized as Targets for IgE Antibodies [Internet]. Available from: http://www.allergen.org/carboep.php)

[31] Lu Y, Sun L, Li C, Wang X, Li W, Zhao T, et al. Comparative mass spectrometry analysis of N-glycans from the glycoproteins of eight allergy-inducing plants. Food Chemistry. 2022;**384**:132440

[32] Platts-Mills TA, Hilger C, Jappe U, van Hage M, Gadermaier G, Spillner E, et al. Carbohydrate epitopes currently recognized as targets for IgE antibodies. Allergy. 2021;**76**(8):2383-2394

[33] Chinuki Y, Morita E. Alpha-Gal-containing biologics and anaphylaxis. Allergology International. 2019;**68**(3):296-300

[34] Nkurunungi G, Mpairwe H, Versteeg SA, Diepen A, Nassuuna J, Kabagenyi J, et al. Cross-reactive carbohydrate determinant-specific IgE obscures true atopy and exhibits α-1,3-fucose epitope-specific inverse associations with asthma. Allergy. 2021;**76**(1):233-246

[35] Jappe U, Schwager C, Schromm AB, González Roldán N, Stein K, Heine H, et al. Lipophilic allergens, different modes of allergen-lipid interaction and their impact on asthma and allergy. Frontiers in Immunology. 2019;**10**:122

[36] Johansson SGO. The discovery of IgE. The Journal of Allergy and Clinical Immunology. 2016;**137**(6):1671-1673

[37] Johansson SGO. Discovery and development of IgE assays. Clinical and Experimental Allergy. 1997;**27**:60-63

[38] van Hage M, Hamsten C, Valenta R. ImmunoCAP assays: Pros and cons in allergology. The Journal of Allergy and Clinical Immunology. 2017;**140**(4):974-977

[39] Jensen-Jarolim E, Jensen AN, Canonica GW. Debates in allergy medicine: Molecular allergy diagnosis with ISAC will replace screenings by skin prick test in the future. World Allergy Organization Journal. 2017;**10**:33

[40] Larenas-Linnemann D, Luna-Pech JA, Mösges R. Debates in Allergy Medicine: Allergy skin testing cannot be replaced by molecular diagnosis in the near future. World Allergy Organization Journal. 2017;**10**(1):32

[41] Valenta R, Campana R, Focke-Tejkl M, Niederberger V. Vaccine development for allergen-specific immunotherapy based on recombinant allergens and synthetic allergen peptides: Lessons from the past and novel mechanisms of action for the future. The Journal of Allergy and Clinical Immunology. 2016;**137**(2):351-357

[42] Egger M, Hauser M, Himly M, Wopfner N, Wallner M, Ferreira F. Development of recombinant allergens for diagnosis and therapy. Frontiers in Bioscience (Elite Edition). 2009;**1**(1):77-90

Chapter 3

Aerobiology in the Clinics of Pollen Allergy

Franziska Zemmer and Fatih Ozkaragoz

Abstract

Diagnosis and treatment of pollen allergies is facilitated by the cooperation between the allergist and the aerobiologist. The selection of relevant allergens for in vivo diagnosis, the interpretation of results, the timing of trials, and treatments should be related to the local pollen season, abiotic variables, and the patient history. Meteorological aspects and flowering dynamics of plants condition the course of the pollen season each year. Pollen forecasting integrates weather data with long- and short-term pollen data. Crowdsourced patient symptoms are used to delineate pollen threshold loads in the forecast. Integrating aerobiological expertise warrants the success of allergy diagnostics and treatment.

Keywords: Pollen allergy, diagnostics, allergenicity, aerobiology, forecasting, pollen thresholds

1. Introduction

With the establishment of skin testing to diagnose for allergy, botanical knowledge on allergenic pollen sources became essential. The synergistic cooperation between allergists and botanists from those years shall be illustrated with an example from Ankara (Turkey), where in 1967 the botanist Kamil Karamanoglu and allergist Kemal Özkaragöz issued lists of allergenic plants, the way their pollen is carried (by wind or insects), their form of growth, and where and in which plant communities they grew [1]. Based on that knowledge, clinical trials were commenced to investigate the allergenic potential of pollen [2] based on the Thommen's postulates [3]. Subsequently, the first Turkish pollen calendar was published for Ankara [4].

Nowadays, pollen information is issued regularly by competent monitoring intuitions as preventive measure for the allergic population in many countries. According to biogeographic peculiarities, the vegetation cover differs from region to region giving rise to varying types of pollen allergens. Which allergens to use in test batteries grounds on the knowledge of the allergenic pollen flora of the area. Immunotherapy, the only treatment that may lead to longer-lasting relief of the burden, can only be successful by considering the geographic circumstances of the patient. That means to work with relevant and good quality pollen data, have information on the course and intensity of the pollen season, and be able to interpret this information. The aerobiologists' point of view on immunotherapy and the implementation of clinical trials has been elaborated, and standards for aerobiological tasks in clinical trials proposed [5].

This to prevent harm to patients, increase the quality and success of the trial, and to obtain comparable results (ibid).

Electronic health technology (eHealth) and mobile applications (mHealth) are, on one hand, a popular way to convey pollen information to the public. Registered users, on the other hand, provide data on their symptoms, which can be used to improve forecasting, monitor public allergy morbidity, and be part of studies on pollen allergy [6]. Pollen threshold loads for symptom development, for example, can be assessed this way along with aerobiological data [7].

In this chapter, we elaborate, firstly, on the allergist's perspective on the choice of allergens, emphasizing the need for diagnostics without harming the patient, and when serum-specific IgE testing is adequate. We delineate limitations of allergy tests and explain why not every pollen type causes an allergic response.

Secondly, we convey the aerobiologist's perspective on pollen forecasting, the role of pollen threshold loads obtained with crowdsourced patient symptoms, and support this with an example from Istanbul.

2. The allergists' perspective

Skin testing has been used to diagnose allergic disorders for more than 50 years. Back in the mid-twentieth century, pricking the skin with a solution of the allergen using a lancet was the only method but today there are several test devices capable of results that are more reliable and reproducible. Skin testing continues to be the main test to confirm an IgE-mediated immunologic reaction. Not only skin testing is the best indicator of the underlying allergic pathology, but it also remains to be the most inexpensive test with rapid results making it practical in office setting. The binding of specific IgE on tissue mast cells to the offending allergen is the unique attribute of skin testing. Alternatively, the patient can be challenged with the allergen by directly applying it to the mucous membranes, nose, bronchi, or even eyes, but the extra advantage of such procedures does not justify the risk and inconvenience. Allergen skin testing has been shown to exhibit reliable correlation with such mucosal challenges [8].

It is crucial, however, that the physician ordering or interpreting these tests be cognizant of the dynamics that can affect the outcome. Some important considerations as to when these tests are indicated and how they should be interpreted are outlined here.

2.1 Choosing the allergens with clinical relevance

Allergy testing without a clear indication or random testing for arbitrarily chosen allergens is not acceptable. The selection of allergens should be determined based on the patient's exposure history and correlated with their symptoms. The relevant allergens should be based on the medical history, age, and the environment, geography of the patient. Knowledge on the average and the course of the pollen seasons of the patient's geography is essential in this regard [9]. The tested allergens should be able to predict and/or confirm the clinical disease.

Most clinicians would order these tests for two main reasons: (1) the planning of avoidance of the allergen and (2) specific immunotherapy. Interdisciplinary collaboration among allergists, aerobiologists, and atmospheric scientists is important to identify the relevant allergens in the environment connecting the time of exposure to symptoms.

2.2 Allergen sensitivity without allergy

The test results should be validated by associating the exposure to allergens under natural conditions or controlled challenges with the particular allergen. There may be skin sensitivity without symptoms which may not have any validity to the current clinical problem of the patient. Routine use of arrays of skin tests or usual annual tests without a definite clinical indication is unwarranted. Nevertheless, some asymptomatic skin sensitization may be a risk factor for future organ sensitivity; hence, some clinicians would still value this coincidental sensitivity to monitor the patient for future development of clinical allergy. In a prospective trial of 15 asymptomatic patients with positive skin prick test to birch, 60% were later reported to develop true clinical allergy [10]. But we must be aware of the cascade effect in medicine which was brilliantly outlined by James Mold [11] referring to the detrimental process that once triggered proceeds to the inevitable conclusion of unnecessary tests, patient and/or physician anxiety ending up with wrong treatments, adverse effects and/or morbidity and not to mention the uneconomic medical expenses. Healthcare providers must guard against the vortex of this domino effect leading to the collision course of such preventable events. End result of such actions are infants being deprived of essential nutrients, needless anxiety for patients and caregivers, inappropriately prescribed more expensive medications possibly leading to antibiotic resistance, etc. Preventing cascade effects should be a part of the education curriculum of physicians and providers. This is not only important in the field of allergy and immunology but all specialties of medicine, especially in the technology era of healthcare services where more is unfortunately considered better.

2.3 Serum-specific IgE testing

In vitro serum IgE testing is sometimes safer than skin testing in patients with cardiovascular disease, or when severe anaphylactic reactions are expected. We also prefer to perform serum in vitro testing for patients who are unable to withhold their antihistamines or other medications interfering with tests. Another common medication that is problematic for skin testing is Omalizumab, which also interferes with many immunoassays, except the ImmunoCAP method, which usually remains accurate [12]. Skin testing on infants less than a year old may be challenging and results may not reflect true sensitivity [13]; thus, we prefer serum-specific IgE tests for infants as young as 6 to 8 weeks of age which only requires capillary blood collection [14].

On the flip side, caution is advised for commercial remote practice laboratories performing such serum tests. Some laboratories bypass the clinician and perform serum IgE tests based on the history submitted by the patients and start immunotherapy according to these ambiguous serum IgE test results. As with the skin tests, the interpretation of specific serum IgE levels require the same meticulous clinical history, physical examination, and, in some instances, challenges with natural or laboratory exposure to allergens. This, obviously, is not the typical practice of commercial laboratories [11]. The serum-specific IgE level per se may not reflect the clinical sensitivity due to the fact that clonality and affinity of the IgE antibody plays a role in translation of serum IgE production to clinically relevant allergic sensitization [15]. Thus, it is important to understand that, although an IgE-mediated immunological response is necessary to develop allergic disease, it is not sufficient.

2.4 Limitations of allergy tests

False-positive allergy test results may occur. Some tree pollens share cross-reactive carbohydrate determinants with other pollens or, for example, honey bee venom [16]. It is also not uncommon for a pollen-sensitive patient to be living in another area, not exposed to the same pollen. The co-sensitization should be differentiated from cross-sensitization when testing with extract reagents with common epitopes. Another reason for getting negative reading on allergy tests is the fact that the pathogenesis of the organ sensitization may not involve IgE-mediated pathways. Alternative immunologic pathways or non-immunologic pathways may be at play. The clinician should be in close contact and consult other specialties as well, to fully understand the scope of the organ symptoms. Also, patients who experienced an anaphylactic event may have false-negative skin test results for up to 2–3 weeks after the episode. In vitro testing serum-specific IgE levels are not affected and can be performed in the post-anaphylactic situation where testing cannot be postponed.

Serum-specific IgE test can also display false-positive or -negative levels based on the binding affinity/avidity of the offending allergen to the solid-phase system used for testing. The circulating levels of cross-reactive peptides and specific antibodies of another class, e.g. IgG or the high levels of nonspecific serum IgE levels, may also affect the readings. We do not perform IgG or IgG subclass antibody tests for food or other allergies. They have no clinical relevance. There have been reports of monitoring IgG4 during venom immunotherapy, but this is not validated [17].

2.5 Not all pollens are created equal

Most pollen types do not cause allergies and the ones that cause allergies do so in different potencies. Not all pollen types elicit an allergic response or in immunologic terms have the recognition moieties, the epitopes, that bind to specific receptors on B or T cells. Allergenicity is usually elicited by the peptidic epitopes. The glycan moieties of these glycoproteins affect the immunogenicity of these peptides. Glycans are in variable proportions in different pollens affecting allergenicity. Even when they do have these epitopes, the conformational shape of the pollen structure may limit the three-dimensional spatial alignment of the allergen to the IgE antibody binding sites. These are some of the factors that will alter the allergenicity of pollen intrinsically at the biochemical level.

Environmental factors also have effects on the allergenicity of pollen. Pollutants such as heavy metals, ozone, sulfur dioxide, nitrogen dioxide, and diesel exhaust particles may affect the allergenicity [18], by activating the immune system, referred to as the adjuvant effect [19]. Extended pollen seasons linked to climate change were recognized as factors for, not only increased pollen production but also increased allergen content of their grains [20, 21].

3. The aerobiologists' perspective

3.1 Forecasting

We see them in newspapers, on weather apps, and on specific pollen apps: warnings on allergenic particles currently airborne in a certain region. Issuing pollen forecasts is the inherent chore of an aerobiologist. Trained technicians count meticulously every pollen grain captured on a slide on a number of vertical or horizontal transects under a light microscope at a magnification of 400 x so to cover at least 10% of the slide's surface to estimate the concentration of airborne pollen per cubic meter air per day [22]. This procedure, where pollen is sampled with a volumetric Hirst-type device on a weekly basis, and evaluated retrospectively, falls under the norm CSN EN 16868 [23]. Issuing warnings based on retrospective data makes forecasting essential. The longer the time series of daily or possibly bi-hourly data, the better will be the forecast. Curves of mean pollen concentrations for each pollen type help to assess the variability within years. For allergy pollen warnings, the aerobiologist uses weather forecasts, past year's data and ideally observes the phenology of plants shedding allergic pollen [24, 25]. Models like SILAM (System for Integrated modeling of Atmospheric composition) [26] and COSMO-ART (Consortium for Small-scale Modeling Aerosols and Reactive Trace gases) [27] can provide additional information to incorporate in pollen warnings in Europe.

3.2 Pollen threshold loads

Although forecasts are useful to help patients avoid exposure when levels are high, pollen and weather data alone do not bear the information, whether or not there is an actual risk for the allergic population to suffer symptoms of allergy. It has been shown that allergy morbidity to a specific pollen type may change over the pollen season [7, 28, 29]. With the inclusion of patient's symptom data, a dose–response relationship between exposure and symptoms can be estimated and the accuracy of pollen load thresholds determined. The focus hereby can be on the allergenic pollen type itself, for example, grasses [28, 30], ragweed [7, 31], or birch [32].

There are several ways to obtain patient symptoms, as reviewed in [33]. Practicable are, for example, questionnaire-based daily surveys for prospective clinical trials [29]. Items may include a four-point symptom scale (0 = zero; 1 = mild; 2 = moderate; and 3 = severe) related to the eyes, nose, bronchi, and medication use [ibid]. Additionally, general health is assessed on a ten-point scale [31]. Study participants may send their data to the research-coordinator daily or weekly. This way to gather symptom data is laborious but allows for the control of missing or hampered data [31]. The number of patients in exposure studies, however, is often limited in size ranging from 12 to 430 in 26 studies as reviewed in a Finnish study [34].

Another way to obtain self-reported patient data on symptoms is by means of electronic pollen diaries. Examples of crowdsourced data include the Dutch Allergieradar.nl, established in 2009 to "improve the hay fever forecasts and to decrease the amount of hay fever symptoms patients experience" [35]. The Europe-wide active pollendiary.com [36] coordinated by the Medical University of Vienna follows the same aim. Pollen data from adhering pollen monitoring networks and single stations are fed into the EAN (European Allergy Network). Registered users are encouraged to log their symptoms regularly over the hay fever period. The service is also available as an application "Pollen" that, as the website, provides personalized symptom forecasts based on previous five records [37]. The application is currently available in Austria, Germany, Switzerland, Sweden, Spain, Great Britain, and South Tyrol [38]. As emphasized in [37], the expertise of the aerobiologist is a pillar to generate personalized pollen information. The symptoms recorded translate into a 3-day allergy risk forecast for the respective region, where a sampling device is located. This personalized forecast includes, besides pollen and weather data, other risk factors for respiratory allergy like ozone, sulfur dioxide, nitrogen dioxide, and particulate matter.

3.3 The power of crowdsourced data

The development of pollendiary.com is a result of yearlong collaboration between a network of aerobiologists, data scientists, and sound management. Quality assurance is a main concern to avoid potential harm to hay fever sufferers due to inaccurate forecasts [39]. An evaluation of nine free applications showed that the accuracy of the grass pollen load forecast was 50% of six apps when compared to the actual grass pollen concentration in the location [39]. Web-based applications are an easy way to self-empower hay fever sufferers and to monitor symptom development in the allergic population. The number of hay fever morbidity data obtained between 2009 and 2019 by means of pollendiary.com across Europe was 240.000, with 190.000 logs from Germany and over 32.000 from Austria [6]. The solid number of crowdsourced data on symptoms enables the aerobiologist to provide more accurate forecasts. As a matter of fact, regional pollen concentrations alone cannot be a measure for the pollen allergenicity experienced by the population in a certain area. It is known that pollen concentrations do not exactly correlate with the allergen content in the air, as shown for ragweed in Turkey [40] or olive in Spain [41]. Pollen potency, the ratio between pollen and allergen concentrations per cubic meter, varies considerably in time and space [42, 43]. The origin of the allergen content in the air is at present not predictable as linked to ruptures of pollen that release micronic allergenic particles at varying weather conditions and altitude, resuspensions, long range transport via air currents, and the allergen content in the plants of origin [42]. Thus, the inclusion of locally experienced symptom data in pollen warnings is essential to issue the correct threshold loads for a particular region.

3.4 An example from Istanbul

The assessment of local thresholds is a pressing issue in allergology [44]. They are unique in each biogeographic area, as factors like pollen sources, their allergenicity, climate, pollution, and the genetic fingerprint at individual and population level are determining factors for symptom thresholds [33]. Crowdsourced symptom data, pollen, weather, and pollution data can be included in models that display the dose–response relationship experienced by the allergic population. Standardized pollen data as in the EAN and a uniform method for symptom data collection as in pollendiary.com allows for the calculation of threshold levels, for example, with nonlinear regression models [7, 45]. Anti-allergic medication can be an indicator for allergy morbidity. Here we show preliminary results of a study conducted with data ($n = 725$) from the European part of Istanbul (**Figure 1**).

In Istanbul anti-allergy medication use started at about 4 p/m^3, and increased linearly till about 11 p/m^3. Subsequently, the bending of the curve [46] suggests that the threshold for moderate medication use has been reached. Between 18 p/m^3 and 30 p/m^3 medication use was the most intense. After that it decreased to remain at a moderate level at >= 50 p/m^3. As few as about 4 p/m^3 caused morbidity that patients sought to mitigate with drugs. In Istanbul the non-linear relationship in the dose-response curve illustrates that symptoms do not necessarily aggravate at a grass pollen concentration higher than 25-30 p/m^3. Longer time series of data with more users than the ones presented here would yield more solid results. Promoting the use of an electronic hay fever symptom diary should be an integral part of a public pollen information system.

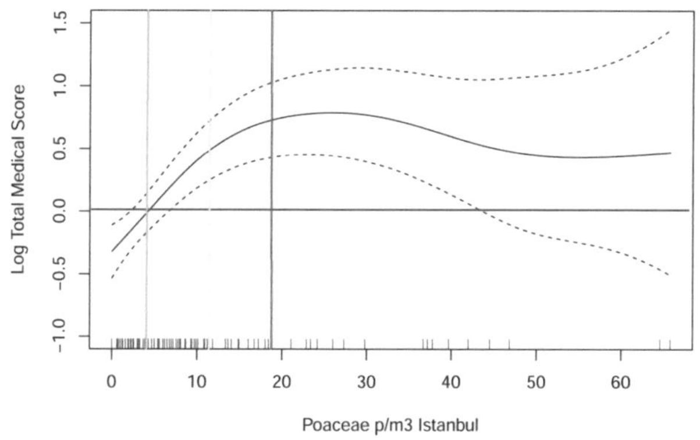

Figure 1.
Preliminary effect curve of pollen concentrations (p/m³) (2014–June 2016) in Istanbul on medication use with thresholds. The green line denotes the start of medication use in unit increase in the log (y) abundance by unit increase in x. The yellow line denotes the threshold for moderate medication use. The red line marks the saturation threshold for intense medication use. The blue line marks zero effect. Note the relationship between the confidence intervals and the data logs.

4. Conclusions

Aerobiological expertise plays an integral role in the clinics of allergic disease in the qualitative forecasting of the pollen season to support the allergist in the assessment of morbidity and the timing of treatment. Cooperation between the allergist and the aerobiologist help select the most relevant allergens for in vivo diagnosis, improve the interpretation of results, and select the most appropriate immunotherapy regimen tailored for the patient.

Acknowledgements

We thank Uwe Berger, MBA from the Aerobiology and Pollen Information Research Unit, Department of Oto-Rhino-Laryngology, Medical University of Vienna, for granting permission to use symptom data from pollendiary.com for the preliminary analysis of pollen thresholds.

Author details

Franziska Zemmer[1*] and Fatih Ozkaragoz[2]

1 Free University of Bolzano, Bolzano, Italy

2 Academic Allergy Asthma and Immunology Assoc, Houston, USA

*Address all correspondence to: franziska.zemmer@unibz.it

References

[1] Karamanoglu K, Özkaragoz K. A preliminary report on the allergenic plants of Ankara. Annals of Allergy. 1967;**25**:23-28

[2] Özkaragöz K. Pollens, mold spores, and other inhalants as etiologic agents of respiratory allergy in the central part of Turkey. Journal of Allergy. 1967;**40**(1):21-25

[3] Thommen AA. Which plants cause hay fever? In: Asthma and Hay Fever in Theory and Practice. Springfield, IL: Charles C. Thomas Publisher; 1931. pp. 546-554

[4] Karamanoglu K, Özkaragöz K. A preliminary study on allergenic pollen producing plants of the Ankara area and their pollination calendar. Review of Palaeobotany and Palynology. 1968;**7**:61-67

[5] Bastl K, Bastl M, Bergmann KC, Berger U. How to do a clinical trial? Recommendations from the aerobiological point of view. World Allergy Organization Journal. 2019;**12**(4):100020

[6] Bastl K, Bastl M, Bergmann KC, Berger M, Berger U. Translating the burden of Pollen allergy into numbers: 10-year observational study of electronically generated symptom data from the patient's Hayfever diary in Austria and Germany. Journal of Medical Internet Research. 2020;**22**(2):e16767

[7] Jones NR, Agnew M, Banic I, Grossi CM, Colón-González FJ, Plavec D, et al. Ragweed pollen and allergic symptoms in children: Results from a three-year longitudinal study. Science of the Total Environment. 2019;**683**:240-248

[8] Bousquet J, Lebel B, Dhivert H, Bataille Y, Martinot B, Michel FB. Nasal challenge with pollen grains, skin-prick tests and specific IgE in patients with grass pollen allergy. Clinical Allergy. 1987;**17**(6):529-536

[9] Zemmer F, Cenk E, Dahl A, Galan C, Ozkaragoz F. A multidisciplinary approach of outdoor aeroallergen selection for skin prick testing in the geographical area of Greater Istanbul. European Annals of Allergy and Clinical Immunology [Internet]. 2021 Jan [cited 2021 Mar 9];(online first). Available from: http://www.eurannallergyimm.com/cont/online-first/914/original-articlebra-multidisciplinary-approach-outdoor-aeroallergen-selection.asp?pgg=1

[10] Bodtger U, Poulsen LK, Malling HJ. Asymptomatic skin sensitization to birch predicts later development of birch pollen allergy in adults: A 3-year follow-up study. The Journal of Allergy and Clinical Immunology. 2003;**111**(1):149-154

[11] Mold JW, Stein HF. The cascade effect in the clinical care of patients. The New England Journal of Medicine. 1986;**314**(8):512-514

[12] Bernstein IL, Li JT, Bernstein DI, Hamilton R, Spector SL, Tan R, et al. Allergy diagnostic testing: An updated practice parameter. Annals of Allergy, Asthma, & Immunology. 2008;**100**(3):S1-S148

[13] Burks AW, editor. Middleton's Allergy: Principles and Practice. Ninth ed. Edinburgh: Elsevier; 2020. p. 2

[14] Hill DJ, Hosking CS, Reyes-Benito LV. Reducing the need for food allergen challenges in young children: A

comparison of *in vitro* with *in vivo* tests: Food allergen challenges in children. Clinical & Experimental Allergy. 2001;**31**(7):1031-1035

[15] Christensen LH, Holm J, Lund G, Riise E, Lund K. Several distinct properties of the IgE repertoire determine effector cell degranulation in response to allergen challenge. The Journal of Allergy and Clinical Immunology. 2008;**122**(2):298-304

[16] Burzyńska M, Piasecka-Kwiatkowska D. A review of honeybee venom allergens and allergenicity. International Journal of Molecular Sciences. 2021;**22**(16):8371

[17] Vanhalteren H, Vanderlinden P, Burgers J, Bartelink A. Discontinuation of yellow jacket venom immunotherapy: Follow-up of 75 patients by means of deliberate sting challenge. The Journal of Allergy and Clinical Immunology. 1997;**100**(6):767-770

[18] Ghiani A, Aina R, Asero R, Bellotto E, Citterio S. Ragweed pollen collected along high-traffic roads shows a higher allergenicity than pollen sampled in vegetated areas. Allergy. 2012;**67**(7):887-894

[19] Gilles S, Behrendt H, Ring J, Traidl-Hoffmann C. The Pollen Enigma: Modulation of the allergic immune response by non-allergenic, pollen-derived compounds. Current Pharmaceutical Design. 2012;**18**(16):2314-2319

[20] Galán C, Thibaudon M. Climate change, airborne pollen, and pollution. Allergy. 2020;**75**(9):2354-2356

[21] Galán C, Garcia-Mozo H, Carinanos P, Alcázar P, Dominguez-Vilches E. The role of temperature in the onset of the Olea europaea L. pollen season in southwestern Spain. International Journal of Biometeorology. 2001;**45**(1):8-12

[22] Galán C, Smith M, Thibaudon M, Frenguelli G, Oteros J, Gehrig R, et al. Pollenmonitoring:Minimumrequirements and reproducibility of analysis. Aerobiologia. 2014;**30**(4):385-395

[23] CEN 16868. Ambient air - Sampling and analysis of airborne pollen grains and fungal spores for networks related to allergy - Volumetric Hirst method. 2019.

[24] Bucher E, Bottarelli L, De Gironimo V, Verardo P, Anelli P, Ivaldi C, et al. POLLnet - Linee guida per il monitoraggio aerobiologico [Internet]. ISPRA; 2017. p. 50. (Manuali e Linee Guida 151; vol. 151). Available from: http://www.pollnet.it/pubblicazioni.asp

[25] Galán C, Cariñanos P, Alcázar P, Domínguez Vilches E. Spanish aerobiology network (REA): Management and quality manual [Internet]. Córdoba: Argos Impresores S.L.; 2007 [cited 2021 Dec 29]. p. 36. Available from: http://www.uco.es›raa›infor_raa›manual_eng

[26] Sofiev M, Siljamo P, Ranta H, Rantio-Lehtimäki A. Towards numerical forecasting of long-range air transport of birch pollen: Theoretical considerations and a feasibility study. International Journal of Biometeorology. 2006;**50**(6):392-402

[27] Vogel H, Pauling A, Vogel B. Numerical simulation of birch pollen dispersion with an operational weather forecast system. International Journal of Biometeorology. 2008;**52**(8):805-814

[28] Caillaud D, Martin S, Segala C, Besancenot JP, Clot B, Thibaudon M. Nonlinear short-term effects of airborne Poaceae levels on hay fever symptoms.

The Journal of Allergy and Clinical Immunology. 2012;**130**(3):812-814.e1

[29] de Weger LA, Beerthuizen T, Gast-Strookman JM, Plas DT, Terreehorst I, Hiemstra PS, et al. Difference in symptom severity between early and late grass pollen season in patients with seasonal allergic rhinitis. Clinical and Translational Allergy. 2011;**1**(1):18

[30] Becker J, Steckling-Muschack N, Mittermeier I, Bergmann KC, Böse-O'Reilly S, Buters J, et al. Threshold values of grass pollen (Poaceae) concentrations and increase in emergency department visits, hospital admissions, drug consumption and allergic symptoms in patients with allergic rhinitis: A systematic review. Aerobiologia. 2021;**37**(4):633-662

[31] Caillaud D, Thibaudon M, Martin S, Ségala C, Besancenot JP, Clot B, et al. Short-term effects of airborne ragweed pollen on clinical symptoms of hay fever in a panel of 30 patients. Journal of Investigational Allergology & Clinical Immunology. 2014;**24**(4):249-256

[32] Caillaud D, Martin S, Segala C, Besancenot JP, Clot B, Thibaudon M. Effects of airborne birch pollen levels on clinical symptoms of seasonal allergic rhinoconjunctivitis. International Archives of Allergy and Immunology. 2014;**163**(1):43-50

[33] de Weger L, Bergmann KC, Rantio-Lehtimäki A, Dahl Å, Buters J, Déchamp C, et al. Impact of Pollen. In: Allergenic pollen: A review of the production, release, distribution and health impacts. Dordrecht New York: Springer; 2013

[34] Kitinoja MA, Hugg TT, Siddika N, Rodriguez Yanez D, Jaakkola MS, Jaakkola JJK. Short-term exposure to pollen and the risk of allergic and asthmatic manifestations: A systematic review and meta-analysis. BMJ Open. 2020;**10**(1):e029069

[35] Environmental Systems Analysis. Allergieradar.nl (Allergy Radar) [Internet]. 2022. Available from: https://www.wur.nl/en/show/Allergieradar.nl-Allergy-Radar.htm

[36] Berger UE, Jäger S, Bergman KC. PHD, the electronic patient's Hayfever diary. European Respiratory Journal. 2011;**38**:3213

[37] Kmenta M, Bastl K, Jäger S, Berger U. Development of personal pollen information—the next generation of pollen information and a step forward for hay fever sufferers. International Journal of Biometeorology. 2014;**58**(8):1721-1726

[38] Keep up to date with the pollen app! [Internet]. pollenwarndienst.at. 2022. Available from: https://www.pollenwarndienst.at/AT/en/free-pollen-app.html

[39] Bastl K, Berger U, Kmenta M. Evaluation of pollen apps forecasts: The need for quality control in an eHealth service. Journal of Medical Internet Research. 2017;**19**(5):e152

[40] Alan Ş, Sarışahin T, Acar Şahin A, Kaplan A, Pınar NM. An assessment of ragweed pollen and allergen loads in an uninvaded area in the Western black sea region of Turkey. Aerobiologia. 2020;**36**:183-195

[41] Galan C, Antunes C, Brandao R, Torres C, Garcia-Mozo H, Caeiro E, et al. Airborne olive pollen counts are not representative of exposure to the major olive allergen Ole e 1. Allergy. 2013;**68**(6):809-812

[42] Tegart LJ, Johnston FH, Borchers Arriagada N, Workman A, Dickinson JL, Green BJ, et al. 'Pollen potency': The relationship between atmospheric pollen counts and allergen exposure. Aerobiologia. 2021;**37**(4):825-841

[43] Buters J, Prank M, Sofiev M, Pusch G, Albertini R, Annesi-Maesano I, et al. Variation of the group 5 grass pollen allergen content of airborne pollen in relation to geographic location and time in season. The Journal of Allergy and Clinical Immunology. 2015;**136**(1):87-95.e6

[44] Ansotegui IJ, Melioli G, Canonica GW, Caraballo L, Villa E, Ebisawa M, et al. IgE allergy diagnostics and other relevant tests in allergy, a World Allergy Organization position paper. World Allergy Organization Journal. 2020;**13**(2):100080

[45] Zemmer F. Istanbul Pollen Allergen Sensitization Study - IPASS [Internet]. [Córdoba]: Còrdoba; 2022. Available from: https://www.uco.es/ucopress/index.php/es/ucopress@uco.es Estudio de sensibilización de alergenos de polen de Estambul

[46] Benedetti A, Abrahamowicz M, Leffondré K, Goldberg MS, Tamblyn R. Using generalized additive models to detect and estimate threshold associations. International Journal of Biostatistics. [Internet. 2009 Jan 16 [cited 2021 Nov 24];**5**(1) Available from: https://www.degruyter.com/document/doi/10.2202/1557-4679.1172/html

Section 3

Food Allergy

Chapter 4

Food Allergies: New Challenges of Our Civilization

Vladimir Klimov, Natalia Cherevko, Natalia Koshkarova and Andrew Klimov

Abstract

People need to eat and digest food, and if they encounter a food allergy it is a real problem. Moreover, some people have a lifelong sensitization to certain products with the threat of anaphylaxis. This chapter considers different aspects of food allergies, allergenicity of dietary allergens, the significance of the gut microbiota and intestinal epithelium integrity, detailed processes of food sensitization, clinical phenotypes and management of food allergies, and, finally, mechanisms of oral tolerance. Fortunately, the gastrointestinal tract possesses robust tolerogenic mechanisms, in particular, the beneficial gut microbiota, as well as the autonomous enteric nervous system, which taken together with the gut immune cells and molecules may be called the enteric neuroimmune system (ENIS). The *dual-allergen exposure hypothesis* postulates that early oral exposure to food allergens induces tolerance, whereas exposure at non-gastrointestinal sites results in food sensitization and allergy development. In addition, a series of food allergic episodes does not look like a typical atopic disease and is a known exception to the rule conceived by evolution. However, the prevalence of food allergies is continuously growing, including severe cases, and it is a paradoxical problem in the face of evolution. This challenge is inherent to our civilization and will be resolved, thanks to new knowledge and technologies.

Keywords: food allergens, enteric neuroimmune system, intestinal epithelium, food sensitization, dual-allergen exposure hypothesis, oral tolerance, AIT

1. Introduction

The term "food allergy" is used to denote an adverse immunologic response to a food protein (allergen) and differ it from so-called "food intolerance" caused by digestive enzyme insufficiency [1]. It is estimated that 3–4% of adults and 5% of children under four years of age in industrialized and westernized countries suffer from food allergies with a broad range of polymorphic signs and symptoms. More extensive data suggest that food allergies account for even up to 10% of affected [2]. The prevalence of food allergies is continuously growing, including severe anaphylaxis caused by selected food allergens like peanuts in separate atopic individuals that can repeat for their lifetime in about 80% of them and maybe fatal [3, 4]. By contrast, food intolerance does not engage the immune system and does not lead to anaphylaxis, but it affects more than half the world's human population.

Nevertheless, a food allergy in isolation does not look like a typical atopic disease and it is rather not a chronic atopic disease but a series of discrete allergic episodes. The gastrointestinal tract is normally a specific target organ unlike the other target organs because food components have to be used for growth and metabolism in children and renewal of the body in adults. Evolution created the gut as a tolerance zone but not a place of immune responses to nutrients. Of course, there is an enormous number of various microbes of the microbiota inhabiting the gut, and the immune system has to control the possible danger of opportunistic microbiota and pathogenic microbes, which can enter the gastrointestinal tract with food. Yet why does the immune system fight against some food proteins that lead to the disease? Undoubtedly, it is a violation of the rules conceived by evolution [5]. However, food allergies are becoming yet another problem for healthcare professionals worldwide. Furthermore, it is accompanied by a buildup of metabolic syndrome, obesity, type 2 diabetes mellitus, and chronic gastrointestinal diseases, which appear to be associated with food expansion, changed dietary behavior and preferences, new food products unknown to human natural history, instability of the gut microbiota, and, possibly, hidden food allergies based on local persistent inflammation in the gut.

Along with global changes on the planet, such as climate change, the loss of biosphere balance, a decrease in species biodiversity, SARS-Cov-2 pandemic and possible new pandemics, threat of vital resources insufficiency required for the survival of mankind, and an increase in the prevalence of food allergies represent a new challenge for our civilization and human evolution.

2. Food allergens and their allergenicity

Food allergens are a small portion among all dietary proteins. The term "allergenicity" describes the characteristic features of food allergens, which enable the sensitization, allergic inflammation, and clinical food allergies.

The well-known "Big Eight" of food allergens exhibits the strongest allergenicity and causes about 90% of all food-allergic cases. The "Big Eight" includes peanut, tree nuts, soy, wheat, cow's milk, hen's eggs, fish, and crustacean shellfish (see **Figure 1**). Allergens in cow's milk, hen's eggs, and wheat often lose their allergenicity when babies grow and acquire allergen tolerance. However, allergies to peanuts, tree nuts, fish, and crustacean and mollusk shellfish usually persist over a lifetime and have a high correlation with anaphylaxis [1, 3, 6].

In total, there are three classes of food allergens.

Class 1 food allergens (cow's milk, peanut, hen's eggs, etc.) are canonical oral allergens that cause sensitization through the gastrointestinal tract and display severe clinical signs.

Class 2 food allergens (e.g., carrot, celery, apple, melon, and kiwi) are cross-reactive dietary allergens with aero-allergens that trigger sensitization through the unified airway and exert less severe cross-reactions termed "oral allergy syndrome" [1, 7].

Class 3 food allergens (e.g., small food proteins less than 10 kDa, additives, contaminants, and colorants like tartrazine) with no capacity of cross-reactivity cause sensitization through the unified airway or skin and frequently result in occupational allergies [8].

DOI: http://dx.doi.org/10.5772/intechopen.106627

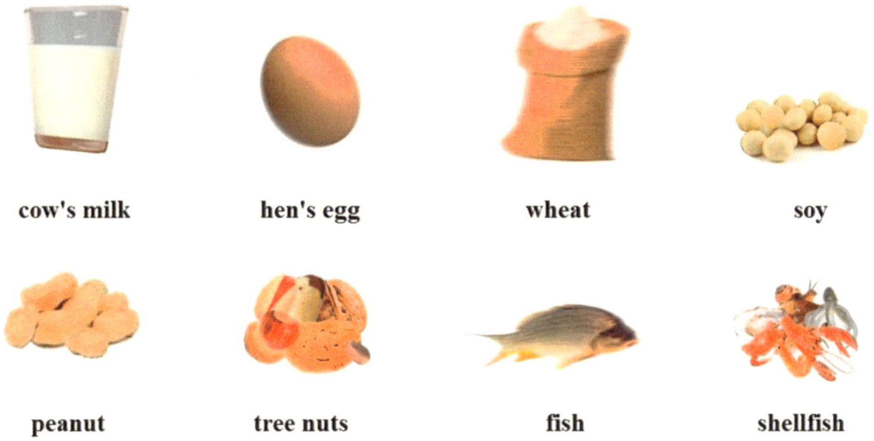

Figure 1.
The "Big Eight" of food allergens. The food allergen group "Big Eight" includes cow's milk, hen's egg, wheat products, soy, peanut, and peanut-containing products, tree nuts, fish, and shellfish. The most frequency of tree nut allergy is attributed to hazelnuts, cashews, pistachios, and almonds. There are many classifications of the shellfish among them we can highlight a division of shellfish into predominant as food allergy triggers crustaceans like shrimps, crabs, and lobster, and slightly less culprit mollusks like oysters, clams, snails, and octopus.

The allergenicity of food nutrients, which are proteins, glyco- or lipoproteins, including novel and genetically modified food ingredients, is evaluated by many techniques such as mass spectrometry, serological assays, cell experiments, animal models, bioinformatics analysis, etc. [9–11].

Factors affecting food protein allergenicity are divided into three groups depending on (1) allergen itself, (2) biogenic cofactors, and (3) the immune system of the body (**Table 1**) [12, 13].

In addition, food allergens generally have to be recognized as heat-stable and heat-labile molecules. Heat-stable allergens are resistant to heat and acid and can cause systemic reactions. In contrast, heat-labile allergens are highly sensitive to heat and acid and may lead to cross-reactivity if they get into the body as pollen particles [14].

The nomenclature of food allergens [15] corresponds to the rules of the established antigen nomenclature, by which the order of letters is as follows: at the beginning, the first three letters of the genus name; next, the first letter of the species name; then the Arabic numeral of when this food allergen was identified among other allergens in this species; and after a period (.), the digits related to isoallergens. For example, an allergen of peanut, *Arachis hypogaea,* may be designated as *Ara h 1.0101.*

In atopic individuals, food allergens induce IgE antibody production by plasma cells due to type 2 helper T (Th2) cell-dependent B-cell adaptive responses, or Th2 pathway. Since 1978 [16] until the present day, the main characterization of allergens, including food allergens, is still defined by their IgE-binding frequency, which enables the division of them into *major* (more than 50% IgE-binding), or *minor* (less than 50% IgE-binding) [17]. However, this classification has become outdated because the new molecular era in allergology has already begun [18]. In the transition period of allergology natural history, two allergen generations are used by allergists for the diagnosis and allergen-specific immunotherapy (AIT):

1. natural standardized allergenic extracts, and.

2. artificial biotechnologically engineered allergenic molecules [17].

Factors of allergen itself	Biogenic cofactors	Factor of the immune system
Primary amino acid sequence of allergenic epitopes; molecular weight lower than 70 kDa; small isoelectric point (charge); degree of protein fold; oligomerization; amount of allergenic epitopes and their proximity to each other; concentration; dose; low hydrophobicity; solubility in water; interaction with lipids; abundance in food; high stability and resistance to the extremes of food processing, denaturation and proteolysis by digestive enzymes; and presence of intrinsic allergen biologic activities	Presence of molecular patterns and adjuvants in food	Hereditary predisposition to atopy; ability to promote the production of elevated levels of high-affinity allergen-specific IgE; route of exposure; involving innate immunity; impaired orogastrointestinal epithelial barrier; influence of the gut microbiota; sialylation of IgE; decreased enzyme secretion; and deficiency in sIgA

Table 1.
Allergenicity factors of food allergens.

The best technique for the determination of specific IgE concentrations produced by food allergens is *component resolved diagnosis (CRD)* [19], which currently exists in three modifications:

1. singleplex assays (ImmunoCAP, Thermo Fisher Scientific/Phadia, Uppsala, Sweden) assess one allergen at a time; they are much cheaper and do not provide potentially unnecessary information [20];

2. multiplex (ImmunoCAP Immuno Solid-phase Allergen Chip [ISAC]) has been the preferred version for the last decade allowing simultaneous determination toward many IgE molecules [20];

3. customized allergen profiles (Euroline; Euroimmun, Lübeck, Germany) are an intermediate option, which combines allergen extracts and a set of the most relevant related allergenic molecules to evaluate the cross-reactivity, genuine sensitization, and risk profile [21].

The CRD enables an increase in the analytic sensitivity and diagnostic specificity and a decrease in potential risks, possible cross-reactivity versus primary specific sensitization. Novel CRD modifications and new technologies for the determination of sensitization are in development.

The *Basophil activation test (BAT)* as a functional assay displays the opportunity to indirectly detect the presence of allergen-specific IgE. After stimulation of blood basophils with an allergen and negative and positive controls, the cells are stained with antibodies linked to a fluorochrome, which allow the visualization of cells and the measurement of biomarkers CD63 and CD203c using a flow cytometer. BAT and the outcome of oral food challenges have a high correlation with food allergies [22, 23].

Skin prick testing (SPT) [24] and the more rarely used *atopy patch tests* [25] keep on being used as *in vivo* methods operated by allergists worldwide. Despite revolutionary and promising molecular methods such as CRD, allergic skin testing has to be considered as an additional, more selective, third-line diagnostic approach reserved for specific cases, such as polysensitized allergies [26].

3. The intestinal barrier and gut microbiota

3.1 The gut epithelium

The gastrointestinal tract normally represents a potent barrier for various harmful substances, allergens, pathogenic microbes, and parasites, and serves as a transit border through which input and output transport of biomolecules, water, and simple chemicals proceeds. The epithelial lining, a one-layer columnar epithelium with microvilli, linked with glycocalyx on the luminal surface contains many cell lineages among which absorptive enterocytes and colonocytes are predominant. The use of transcriptomic technology, single-cell RNA-sequencing, enabled a revisal of gut epithelium structure and description of the full landscape of cell lineages among conventional cell types (see **Figure 2**) [27, 28].

Absorptive early, intermediate, and mature (1) gut epitheliocytes and (2) intestinal stem cells are reported to be the most numerous, whereas interepithelial (IEC) cells such as (3) transit amplifying cells, (4) bastophin 4 (BEST4+)-positive epitheliocytes, and (5) goblet cells, are shown to be in medium quantities. The remaining IEC, (6) Paneth cells, (7) tuft cells, (8) enteroendocrine (EEC) cells, (9) M cells, and (10) intraepithelial lymphocytes are identified as rare and very rare cell lineages [27, 29].

Functions of gut epitheliocytes include well-regulated absorption of nutrients and water and the barrier obstacle formation for its own microbiota, pathogenic microbes, and allergens due to adhesive interepithelial complexes composed of desmosomes, adherens junctions, and tight junctions [30]. Some known proteins, claudin, aquaporin, aquaglyceroporin provide these epitheliocyte functions [27]. Almost every week, a new epitheliocyte regenerates from stem cells in-built in the epithelial monolayer. However, cells of the epithelium can become a "gate" for food allergens and contribute to allergic inflammation. There are four routes for allergen uptake and entry into the submucosa [29]:

1. paracellular transport of allergen due to epithelium leak;

2. allergen transcytosis by M cells;

3. goblet cell-associated allergen passages (GAP);

4. direct luminal allergen uptake by long outgrowths of dendritic (DC) cells;

The simple columnar intestinal epithelium is well suited for dietary allergen delivery through GAPs since it enables fast access for allergens in a direct manner to lamina propria DCs [31]. In addition, epitheliocytes (1) constitutively express the low-affinity FcεRII (CD23) by which allergens can transcytose via the epithelium in the submucosa [29], and (2) express the pattern recognition receptors (PRR) like

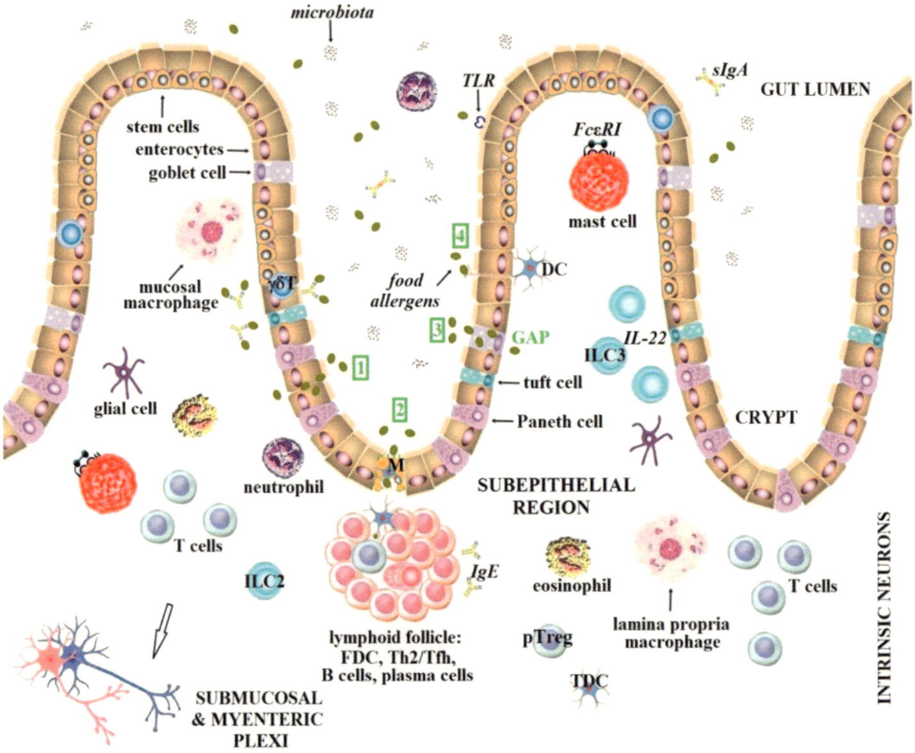

Figure 2.
The gut epithelium and subepithelial region. The gut epithelium landscape is currently revised due to new transcriptomic technology, the single-cell RNA-sequencing. Absorptive enterocytes in the small intestine and colonocytes in the large intestine are prevalent cell lineages. In total, the gut epithelium consists of epitheliocytes and stem cells, and many interepithelial cells perform the main function to protect the subepithelial region and internal environment against invaders and allergens. However, under certain conditions, food allergens can penetrate the epithelial barrier using one or some of four routes: (1) due to impaired epithelium integrity or leak; (2) via specialized M cells; (3) by GAP; and (4) due to uptake by long dendrites of DC. GAP—goblet cell-associated allergen passage, DC—dendritic cell, Th2—type 2 helper T cell, Tfh—follicular dendritic cell, FDC—follicular dendritic cell, ILC2, and ILC3—group 2 and group 3 innate lymphoid cells, TDC—tolerogenic dendritic cell, pTreg—peripheral regulatory T cell, TLR—Toll-like receptors.

Toll-like receptors (TLRs) sensing food allergens and allergen-associated molecular patterns (AAMP) [32, 33].

BEST4+ epitheliocytes, a new cell lineage, are just identified [27]. Enhanced BEST4 expression on BEST4+ epitheliocytes appears to be associated with dietary consumption of sugar and fat [27].

Goblet cells, a predominant cell lineage among IECs, related to secretory cells, are the primary contributor to an additional obstacle for undesirable invaders before the epithelial barrier by secretion of high-molecular-weight glycoprotein complexes [27, 34]. In addition, they promote the process of GAP formation [35], while the GAP function may be present at other mucosal sites different from the gut. Intestinal goblet cells can perform a critical role in the capture of luminal allergens due to the GAP formation [29]. Interestingly, during interactions with DCs, goblet cells transfer these dietary allergens to DCs, which may, conversely, acquire opposite tolerogenic properties becoming tolerogenic CD103+ DCs and taking part in the proliferation of peripheral regulatory T (pTreg) cells [29, 31].

Paneth cells are rare, well-characterized columnar secretory cells, mainly located at the base of the small intestine crypts. In gut inflammation, they have also been revealed within the stomach and colon epithelium. The paneth cells release from their acidophilic granules many antimicrobial factors of neutrophil-like profile, such as α-defensins, lysozyme, IL-1β, IL-17A, TNF, etc., to provide the crypts with a sterile condition, control intestinal microbiota, and contribute to the inflammatory process [36]. The paneth cells have not yet been reported to play a role in food allergies, however, an indirect effect, through the luminal microbiota, which is regulated by these cells, is possible [29].

Tuft cells are less well studied in comparison with other ILCs. Tuft cells are able to be overactivated in relation to helminth and protist invasion, take part in promoting group 2 innate lymphoid (ILC2) cells and Th2 pathway, recognize pathogen-associated molecular patterns (PAMP) via expressed TLRs, and secrete acetylcholine, IL-25, eicosanoids, enzymes, etc. [27, 29, 37]. The ability of tuft cells to communicate with neurons is a subject for future research. There is minimal evidence for their role in food allergies, including the direct effect on food-induced anaphylaxis [29].

EECs produce over 30 neuropeptides, such as calcitonin-gene-related peptide (CGRP), vasoactive intestinal peptide (VIP), substance P, and gastrointestinal hormones [38, 39], which operate not only within the gut but communicate in the gut-brain axis [27]. Neuropeptide W secreted by EEC is known to upregulate food intake [28]. So far, there is no evidence of a functional link between EECs and IgE-mediated food allergies [29].

"Microfold" (M) cells are localized to the lymphoid follicle-covered epithelium and specialized for the uptake of particulate allergens from the lumen facilitating transcellular transport to DCs for allergen processing, allergen uploading on Class II HLA molecule grooves, and presenting to lymphocytes [27, 29, 30]. Taking into consideration the main function of M cells, it is obvious that M cells may perform an essential role in the immunopathogenesis of food allergies [29].

Conventional dendritic cells 2 (DC2s) of which outgrowths pass through the intestinal epithelium can show different phenotypes [29, 40]. At least, some of them exhibit protolerogenic properties to promote pTregs differentiation, which is important for oral tolerance. So far, in the gut, DC subsets are still insufficiently studied in humans, therefore, this information mainly comes from mouse models.

Intraepithelial lymphocytes are CD8αα + γδT cells promoting allergen transcytosis when allergens are complexed with FcεRII (CD23) expressed by epitheliocytes to get into the subepithelial region [29, 41].

3.2 The gut subepithelial region

The underlying mucosal immune system's cells are located in the lamina propria, compressible, and elastic region, where the nourishment and functioning of the epithelium and containing immune cells, nerve fibers, glial cells, and other cells take place (see **Figure 2**).

Peyer's patches, isolated follicles, and the appendix are lymphoid aggregates of the intestine, whereas the scattered lymphoid elements not organized in similar aggregates are available in the esophagus and stomach. In the aggregated lymphoid follicles, there are B-cell areas where follicular dendritic (FDCs) cells and follicular helper T (Tfh) cells promote advanced B-cell-mediated immune response. Plasma cells produce end-products: secretory IgA (sIgA), IgG, and IgE if sensitization occurs. Some allergen-specific DCs migrate via draining lymphatics to mesenteric lymph nodes, where they also trigger advanced B-cell-mediated responses. T-cells are disposed outside the lymphoid follicles in so-called T-cell zones [5].

Cell types of the subepithelial region in addition to those mentioned above are as follows: (1) DC subsets like conventional (myeloid) dendritic (cDC) cells subdivided into cDC1 and cDC2, plasmacytoid dendritic (pDC) cells, tolerogenic dendritic (TDC) cells, and inflammatory dendritic cells, (2) ILC2 and ILC3, (3) mucosal, Peyer's patch, lamina propria, and muscular macrophages (M2), (4) mast cells and basophils, (5) eosinophils, (6) neutrophils, (7) enteric glial cells, (8) fibroblasts, and other cells.

TDCs express integrin α_E (CD103+), complexed with molecule β_7 to form $\alpha_E\beta_7$ receptor for E-cadherin and essential for homing of new T cells in the gut and then to draining lymph nodes to promote pTregs differentiation [42, 43]. They also express integrin $\alpha_4\beta_7$. The inflammatory DC subset generated from monocytes participates in many types of inflammatory processes, including allergic inflammation [44].

ILC2 and ILC3 are located in the submucosa in separation. ILC2 is known as cell activated by epitheliocyte-derived alarmins and neuromedin U and those take part in forwarding the Th2 pathway and allergic inflammation [45]. ILC3, which is more heterogeneous, activated by glial cells and VIP maintains the gut epithelium integrity due to IL-22, as well as regulates lymphoid follicle formation and oral tolerance [46].

Mucosal macrophages (M2) located close to epithelium are responsible for the survival and differentiation of epitheliocytes, intestinal stem cells, and IECs, preservation of epithelial barrier integrity, repair in its disruption, and surveillance for the gut microbiota. The other macrophage subtypes, lamina propria macrophages, Peyer's patch macrophages, and muscular macrophages related to M2 phenotype suppress all potential immune responses [4, 47].

Mast cells are leading cells of allergic inflammation. They are heterogeneous and exist as three mast cell subsets: cells expressing tryptase and chymase (MC_{TC}, or "connective-tissue" cells), mast cells expressing only tryptase (MC_T, or "atypical, or mucosal" cells), and the rare mast cells expressing only chymase (MC_C) [48]. Food allergen binds to produce IgE antibodies, which interact with FcεRI on mucosal mast cells. Mast cells respond, increasing the fluid secretion, smooth muscle contraction, peristalsis, vomiting, and diarrhea due to three portions of pro-inflammatory mediators. There is also the IgE-independent alternative activation pathway of mast cells provided through the Mas-related G-protein-coupled receptor—MRGPRX2 [49]. It leads to the same effects as classical pathway.

Basophils and mast cells share the capacity of degranulating in a rapid manner and releasing histamine, but they differ in their precursors, the ability to synthesize inflammatory eicosanoids, and a particular set of cytokines and chemokines [50]. Mast cells and basophils are upregulated by IL-9 and IL-33 [51]. During recent years, new research facts concerning non-canonical functions of mast cells are accumulated, for example, participation in extracellular trapping, communication with the CNS, and less understood roles in tumorigenesis [50].

Eosinophils, analogous to mast cells, are related to main cells of allergic inflammation [52]. However, eosinophils and IL-5 likely play not such significant roles in food allergies in comparison with allergic inflammatory processes in different target organs [23, 53]. However, eosinophils are undoubtedly leading cells in another separate allergic pathology, eosinophilic esophagitis [54]. The cells have two types of granules, primary and specific/crystalloid, which contain galectin 10 (Charcot-Leyden crystals), major basic protein, eosinophilic cationic protein, eosinophilic peroxidase, enzymes, cysteinyl leukotrienes, histaminase, etc. Most of these factors release during degranulation, affect parasites in a toxic manner, and participate in allergic inflammation [55].

Neutrophils, a prevalent cell lineage among leukocytes, have long been underestimated as cells, which actively participate in allergic inflammation during the late phase [56]. They contain 200 granules of three types, larger azurophilic, smaller specific, and tertiary granules rich in a large number of pro-inflammatory mediators. In allergic asthma the Th2-low/Th17/neutrophylic endotype has been already identified, but, in food allergies, it must be described in the near future because the gut is not only a tolerance zone but the barrier target organ that is a deterrent border for a huge amount of various luminal microbes.

Enteric glial cells modulate the interactions between neurons and the immune system and maintain along with ILC3 the epithelial barrier integrity [57, 58]. Glial cells appear to orchestrate the mutual enteric neuroimmune system (ENIS).

3.3 The gut microbiota

Starting at delivery, then during childhood and all lifetime, microbiota, or microbiome, settles the gut and other barrier organs, changes its composition depending on the microenvironment, and continuously affects vital processes, preventing or promoting pathologic conditions. In this regard, microbiota is heterogeneous and can be divided into two large groups, a beneficial tolerogenic (immunoregulatory) microbiota and potentially harmful inflammatory opportunistic microbiota [59]. The tolerogenic microbiota fulfills dietary fiber fermentation and produces seven short-chain fatty acids: butyrate, propionate, acetate, formate, isobutyrate, valerate, and isovalerate, which are essential factors along with pro-tolerogenic neurotransmitters and neuropeptides for the proliferation and maturation of TDCs and pTreg cells and for the enterocytes and colonocytes regeneration due to the renewal of intestinal stem cells and inhibition of the Th1, Th2 and Th17 lymphocytes activity [60, 61]. Interestingly, the many bacteria of the first group synthesize neuro molecules, serotonin, GABA, opioids, dopamine, required for the immunoregulation in the gut and interaction with the immune and nervous systems [62, 63]. Conversely, inflammatory microbes are prone to promote the maturation of Th1 and Th17, share features with both pathogens and symbionts, and cause pathological processes under particular conditions. These two groups antagonize with each other and compete for nutrients; therefore, the role of the immune system is complex and maybe even paradoxical because it has to provide a differential approach to the gut microbiota.

Tolerogenic microbiota must meet the following criteria [5]:

1. producing metabolites that promote the allergen tolerance maintenance system at the level of the whole body at all times,
2. antagonizing with the other microbes, which may cause gastrointestinal inflammation and food allergies, and
3. dynamic, positive changes depending on the flux microenvironment.

In children, the gastrointestinal tract's immaturity may play a role in the increased prevalence of gastrointestinal dysbiosis and food allergies seen in the first four years of life. In general, in children and adults, the main function of the gastrointestinal tract is to process ingested food into a form that can be absorbed and exploited for energy and growth, and simultaneously prevent the multiplication of undesirable microbiota in the gut. The intake of food proteins normally enables the local and systemic immune unresponsiveness in a process termed oral tolerance [2]. Dysbiosis in children is promoted by unfavorable factors, such as cesarean delivery, lack of breastfeeding, early-life-antibiotic exposure, and a low-fiber/high-fat diet. Allergen tolerance breakdown may be the end-effect of dysbiosis [64]. Adults develop dysbiosis due to diseases, genetic and epigenetic background, unhealthy diet, including a decrease in dietary fibers, vitamins, trace elements, and an increase in fat, sugar, and salt, use of junk foods, tobacco, and alcohol, as well as unhealthy lifestyle, lack of environmental sanitation, immobility, etc.

The communities of microbes comprising the gut microbiota are complex and dynamic from birth to adulthood. Factors affecting the diversity and growth of the gut microbiota show that the microbiota can dramatically influence the outcome of immune responses in the gut, including penetration of food peptides (allergens). Furthermore, this circumstance appears to be the leading cause of IgE-dependent food allergies to start or not [29, 65]. The tolerogenic microbiota is, on the other hand, a strong factor in oral tolerance maintenance at any age [66–69]. However, the ratio of continuous tolerance versus food allergy episodes remains disputable, particularly why most individuals do not get sensitized during their lifetime at all [70].

In non-atopic adults, the IgE-dependent food allergies must not occur, but IgG-mediated food allergies may appear at any age if gastrointestinal disorders are available. There are also food allergic reactions, the previously so-called "*pseudo allergy*." IgE-mediated food allergic reactions may present in different tissues, such as skin, gastrointestinal, respiratory and genitourinary tracts, and allergens penetrate the body in the same ways [1, 23]. However, there is not yet a full clarification why food allergies occur in only some atopic persons but not in all.

4. Enteric neuroimmune system (ENIS)

The gastrointestinal tract is a container of processing food components, digestive enzymes, metabolites, enormous microbiota, immune cells, neurons, glial cells, and immune- and neuron-derived molecules [5].

The gut is innervated by three types of peripheral nervous system counterparts under the general regulation of the central nervous system (CNS): (1) the somatosensory nervous system, (2) the vegetative nervous system subdivided into (i) sympathetic and (ii) parasympathetic divisions, and (3) the unique self-contained nervous system, termed the enteric nervous system (ENS) [71].

Sympathetic innervation of the gut is provided by efferent neurons, which are present in the cut-associated lymphoid (GALT) tissue, and act through β_2ARs expressed on most immune cells secreting preferentially protolerogenic neurotransmitter norepinephrine (NE). In the gastrointestinal tract, norepinephrine diminishes enzyme secretion, food digestion, ENS activity, gut motility, and peristalsis.

Parasympathetic innervation of the gut is achieved with cholinergic neurons, which operate using preferable pro-immunogenic neurotransmitter acetylcholine (ACh) via a7nAchRs expressed on the epithelium's cells and immune cells, promoting the gut inflammatory process, mucus secretion by goblet and other secretory cells, and intestinal peristalsis. However, acetylcholine enables re-switching via vagus-splenic synapse with the sympathetic nervous system and displays temporary pro-tolerogenic activity termed the cholinergic anti-inflammatory pathway [72]. Notably, cholinergic preganglionic-postganglionic neuron synapses are located in ganglia placed in close proximity to the innervated intestine, whereas adrenergic preganglionic fibers form synapses with postganglionic fibers in the symphathetic trunk ganglia [57]. Both sympathetic and parasympathetic neurons are extrinsic for the ENS because their cell bodies reside in the ganglia outside the gut. The sensory fibers of the somatosensory nervous system are mainly carried by the vagus nerve [73], the major parasympathetic nerve.

The ENS is closely linked with the immune system representing, in fact, the mutual enteric neuroimmune system (ENIS). In terms of evolution, ENIS is committed to implement some vital functions, in part controversial, but strictly required for human life as follows:

- food intake, digestion, and nutrient absorption for engagement in metabolic processes in the body;
- cooperation with the gut tolerogenic microbiota and maintenance of its constancy;
- containment of the inflammatory microbiota if re-activated;
- defense against pathogenic microbes entering with food;
- autoimmune and allergen tolerance maintenance;
- preservation of intestinal epithelium integrity and control of its permeability;
- synthesis of cytokines, chemokines, growth factors, neuro molecules, hormones, vitamins, etc.;
- output of feedback signals to the CNS;
- clearance of the body.

The ENIS is composed of a huge number of intrinsic neurons and interneurons, structured in two plexuses, submucosal (disposed between the circular muscle layer and epithelium) and myenteric (located between the longitudinal and circular muscle layers), non-neuronal cells like glia, and neuro molecules affecting the gut and gut functions [57, 58, 73]. Submucosal plexus neurons control gut secretions, food component absorption, and local blood flow, whereas myenteric plexus neurons modulate smooth muscle effects [57, 58]. The ENS, immune cells, and intestinal microbiota secrete many neurotransmitters and neuropeptides among which NE, ACh, serotonin, dopamine, GABA, CGRP, [74, 75], as well as VIP, substance P, and neuromedin U (NMU) are the most significant for the gut (see **Table 2** and **Figure 3**) [76].

Neurotransmitters and neuropeptides serve as the main instrument by which the ENIS controls the homeostasis and all functions in the gut. As you can see in **Table 2**, neuro molecules are presented as predominantly protolerogenic or predominantly pro-immunogenic, and some of them can exert ambivalent activity. In healthy conditions, the summarized potential of neurotransmitters and neuropeptides in the gut is protolerogenic and anti-inflammatory, but in food allergies, conversely,

Neurotransmitters and neuropeptides	Some receptors	Origin source	Prevalent activity in relation to oral tolerance	References
Norepinephrine (NE)	β_2AR; αAR	Sympathetic neurons, adrenal medulla, lymphocytes, NK cells, monocytes, macrophages, EEC	Protolerogenic neurotransmitter	[57, 58, 73, 74, 76–79]
Acetylcholine (ACh)	a7nAchR; M1AchR-M4AchR	Parasympathetic neurons, EEC, lymphocytes, monocytes	Pro-immunogenic neurotransmitter	[57, 71, 76, 78, 80]
Serotonin (5-hydroxytryptamine)	5-HT_1-5-HT_7	Central and enteric neurons, enterochromaffin tissue, EEC	Protolerogenic neurotransmitter	[72, 74, 77, 81, 82]
Dopamine	D_1-D_5	Sympathetic neurons, lymphocytes, DCs, macrophages, neutrophils	Predominantly pro-immunogenic neurotransmitter as well as can exert protolerogenic activity	[72, 74, 77]
γ Aminobutyric acid (GABA)	$GABA_A$-$GABA_B$	Neurons, T cells, macrophages, EEC	Protolerogenic neurotransmitter	[74, 77]
Calcitonin-gene-related peptide (CGRP)	CLRs	Sensory neurons, T cells, B cells, EEC, the thyroid gland	Predominantly protolerogenic neuropeptide as well as can exert ambivalent activity	[57, 71, 76–79]
Vasoactive intestinal peptide (VIP)	VPAC1-VPAC2	Parasympathetic sensory neurons, EEC, the gut	Predominantly protolerogenic neuropeptide as well as can exert ambivalent activity	[57, 58, 71, 73, 76–79, 83]
Substance P	NK1R-NK3R	Sensory neurons, microglia, lymphocytes, DCs, macrophages, eosinophils	Pro-immunogenic neuropeptide	[57, 72, 78, 79]
Neuromedin U (NMU)	NMUR1-NMUR2	Parasympathetic sensory neurons, EEC	Pro-immunogenic neuropeptide	[57, 58, 73, 76, 78, 79]

Table 2.
The most significant neurotransmitters and neuropeptides in the gut.

it is prone to allergen tolerance breakdown and allergic inflammation [5]. Some facts of how neuro molecules influence the human immune cells in the gut allergic inflammatory process are continuously accumulated. However, our knowledge of neuronal-gut immune cell units as a new neuroimmunology paradigm comes mainly from mouse models [58, 84].

NE inhibits ILC2 activity, Th2 pathway [57, 73, 76, 78], and induces anti-inflammatory M2 phenotype of muscular macrophages [58, 73, 74].

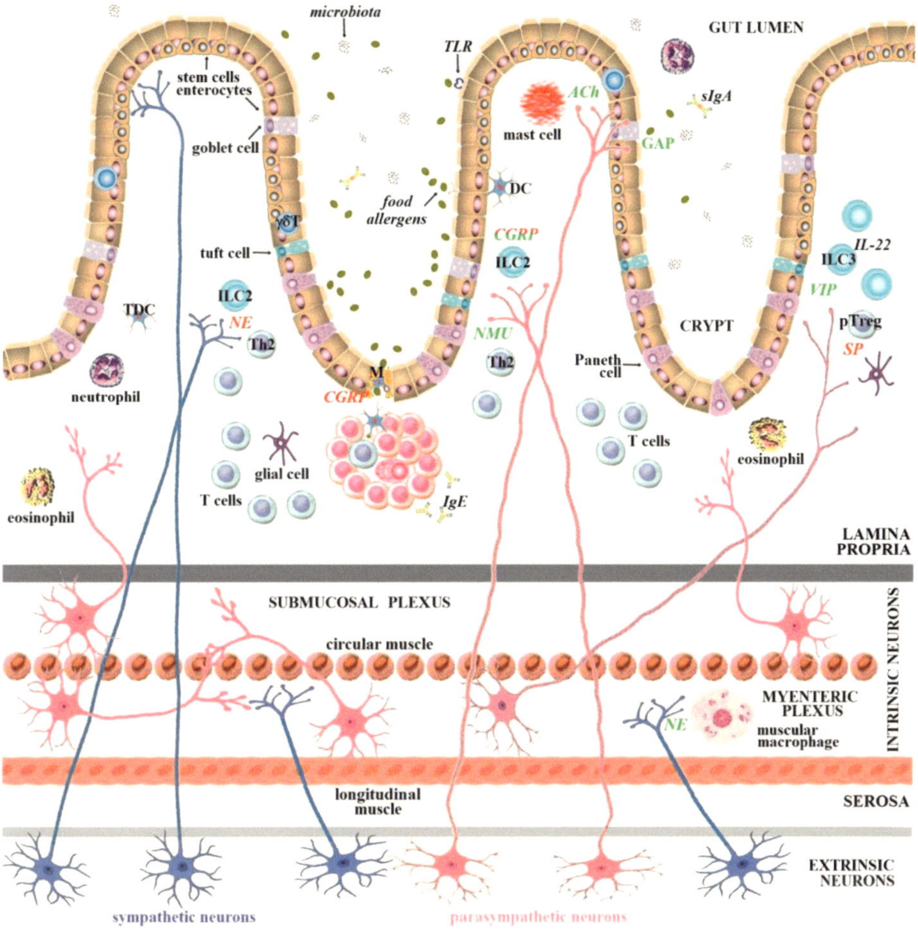

Figure 3.
Enteric neuroimmune system (ENIS). The ENS as a part of combined ENIS forms two plexi, submucosal and myenteric, and contains intrinsic neurons and nerve fibers of sympathetic, parasympathetic, and somatosensory nervous systems of which cell bodies are located outside the ENS. Most sensory fibers are carried by the parasympathetic fibers. Some secreted in the ENIS neuro molecules exert pro-immunogenic effects, in particular, ACh upregulates mucus production, GAP formation, and mast cell degranulation; SP inhibits pTreg proliferation; NMU triggers ILC2 activation and Th2 pathway. In contrast, NE displays protolerogenic activity downregulating ILC2 and Th2 cells, and upregulating M2 polarization of muscular macrophages. CGRP and VIP show ambivalent and even paradoxical effects, for example, CGRP acts on ILC2 in a controversial manner concerning cytokine production, but downregulates M cell development. VIP promotes Th2 pathway and, simultaneously, pTreg cell proliferation and along with glial cells epithelium integrity. ENIS—enteric neuroimmune system, ENS—enteric nervous system, ACh—acetylcholine, SP—substance P, NMU—neuromedin U, NE—norepinephrine, CGRP—calcitonin-gene-related peptide, VIP—vasoactive intestinal peptide, GAP—goblet cell-associated allergen passage, DC—dendritic cell, Th2—type 2 helper T cell, ILC2 and ILC3—group 2 and group 3 innate lymphoid cells, pTreg—peripheral regulatory T cell, TLR—Toll-like receptors. Pro-immunogenic effects are noted in green, and protolerogenic effects are noted in red.

ACh causes goblet cells to secrete mucus, form GAP [76] and amplifies the degranulation of mast cells [80].

Glial cells via neurotrophic factors cause ILC3 to produce IL-22 for the maintenance of the gut epithelium integrity [57, 58].

CGRP acts on ILC2 in a paradoxical manner inhibiting IL-13 secretion and activating IL-4 synthesis [76], but, in total, CGRP downregulates Th2 pathway of immune response responsible for allergic inflammation in the gut [79], including CGRP effect due to M cell downregulation [76].

VIP stimulates IL-22 production by ILC3 [76], and proliferation of pTregs [83], but, on the other hand, promotes Th2 pathway, migration, and survival of Th2 cells [78, 83].

SP upregulates DCs migration, Th1 pathway [72], and inhibits pTreg proliferation in the gut [79].

NMU activates ILC2 and causes them to produce IL-5 and IL-13 [73, 76, 79] that upregulates Th2 pathway of immune response and allergic inflammation.

Most mechanisms of allergic inflammation cannot be explained only by the participation of immune cells and immune-derived molecules. Food allergies are such a case. Since allergic inflammation disrupts homeostasis not only in the gut and other target organs but also in the whole body, neuronal control is extremely necessary. Neuro molecules produced by neurons and non-neuronal cells display short-term life but long-term effects in relation to a place of allergic inflammation and beyond. So far, although numerous studies of neuroimmune interactions in food allergies are the subject of discussion, our comprehension is still incomplete. Taking into account the significance of the subject, this knowledge may become a novel source of updated therapeutic approaches to food allergies in the near future.

5. Sensitization to food allergens and allergic inflammation

There are oral, skin, and respiratory routes of entry of environmental allergens, including food allergens, into the body [1]. Although modern experimental and clinical studies support a role for skin exposure to dietary allergens, which initiate the sensitization and initiation of the Th2 pathway B-cell response, the oral route remains important for food allergies [30].

Experimental studies are reported to highlight the significant role of IECs in the facilitation of dietary allergens to penetrate the epithelial barrier and trigger IgE sensitization [30]. When allergens appear in front of the epithelium, they use any of four transcytosis routes (see **Figure 2** in unit 3) [29] to get into the subepithelial region rich in various cells, including those required for triggering allergic responses. Accordingly, the gut epitheliocytes generate as a "danger signal" particular cytokines called alarmins, IL-25, IL-33, and thymic stromal lymphopoietin (TSLP), upregulating three types of cells: ILC2, allergen-presenting DCs, and Th2 cells. Activated ILC2 produces IL-5, IL-9, and IL-13 influencing over eosinophils and mast cells. Food allergens are engulfed by DCs, processed, uploaded on class II HLA molecule grooves, and as allergen/HLA II complexes presented to lymphocytes, which are activated after recognition and involved in clonal expansion and maturation. Differentiated Th2 cells upregulate the Th2-mediated B-cell response with IgE end-production and memory B and memory T cells formation [3]. Memory about the current allergen becomes lifelong. The whole process proceeds in the lymphoid follicles as well as draining lymph nodes. Interestingly, intestinal epitheliocytes can constitutively turn into allergen-presenting cells like DCs and present allergens to lymphocytes [23].

Th2 pathway activation is called "the type 2 cytokine storm," which stimulates expansion of the main cells of allergic inflammation, mainly mast cells and basophils. Th2 cells produce IL-4, IL-5, IL-9, IL-13, and IL-33, which promote allergic inflammation. Notably, IL-5 does not play a leading role in food sensitization, in contrast to responses to other allergens, in distinct target organs [23]. IL-33 is reported to be essential for the maturation of mast cells [51]. Another immunoregulatory T-cell subset, Tfh cells, secretes IL-21, IL-4, and IL-13, important for IgE class switching due to recombination and somatic mutations in B cells, maturing plasma cells and growing allergen-specific IgE affinity. The degree of involvement of Th9 cells in food sensitization is disputed [85].

Since protolerogenic neurotransmitters and neuropeptides are prevalent in the ENIS, food allergens cannot easily overcome the system of allergen tolerance maintenance. However, if it occurs, allergic inflammation commences, and clinical food allergies develop [5].

Allergic inflammation is an immunopathological process, which proceeds in three phases: (1) early phase, (2) late phase, and (3) chronic allergic inflammation [56]. The *early phase* usually gets started within 2–3 h after uptake of a causative food allergen depending on absorption in the gut or less if in the oral cavity and includes the release of normally preformed mediators of mast cells [50] and basophils, such as histamine, serotonin, chemotactic peptides for neutrophils and eosinophils, and enzymes (chymase and tryptase). These mediators affect the nerve cells causing smooth muscle contraction, mucus production by goblet cells, increased capillary permeability, recruitment of neutrophils and eosinophils. In some cases, mast cells release a wide range of chemicals in greater quantity than usual, causing reactions collectively known as anaphylaxis in multiple body areas, including the unified airway, cardiovascular system, brain, etc. Frequently, it may be a life-threatening condition [86].

The *late phase* in food allergies develops in 6–9 h and later. Two groups *de novo* produced after activation of mast cells and basophils neoformed and neosynthesized mediators consist of cysteinyl leukotrienes (LTC_4, LTD_4, and LTE_4), prostaglandin D_2 (PGD_2), platelet-activating factor (PAF), pro-inflammatory cytokines, chemokines, growth factors, nitric oxide, and C3 and C5 components of complement [87]. These biomolecules act on surrounding tissues promoting the inflammatory process. Endothelial cells express those adhesion molecules, which facilitate the involvement and activation of neutrophils, eosinophils, inflammatory DCs, and monocytes from the blood into the site of the allergic inflammation. The eosinophils release various inflammatory molecules, including major basic protein, eosinophilic cationic protein, IL-5, etc. The involved Th2 cells secrete cytokines among which Il-4, IL-13, and IL-33 are the most potent and affect plasma cells, promoting IgE isotype switching. So, the events acquire long-term potential [5].

The process becomes *chronic allergic inflammation* after repeated exposures to food allergens and continuous recruitment of inflammatory cells releasing numerous pro-inflammatory mediators. In food allergies, in the gut, local persistent allergic inflammation is inherent though clinical signs may manifest only from time to time.

6. Food allergies as particular atopic conditions

The natural history of food allergies contains attempts to explain why this type of allergy occurs. Some hypotheses have been proposed and are still being discussed [2, 88].

The hygiene hypothesis and "old friends" hypothesis. The absence of exposure to microbes and allergens in early childhood may increase predisposition to allergic sensitization due to the underdevelopment of the immune system promoting Th2 polarization rather than Th1.

The dual-allergen exposure hypothesis. In infants, if the skin barrier function is impaired, exposure to environmental food allergens causes allergen sensitization through the skin rather than via oral route. Food allergies are likely generated as a combination of both skin and gut exposure to food allergens, with a preferable tendency towards sensitization through the skin route. Proponents of the hypothesis attempt to put the idea of early introduction of allergenic food for susceptible babies into practice [6, 89].

The vitamin D hypothesis. Vitamin D (cholecalciferol) is a recognized immunomodulatory and protolerogenic substance of which deficiency may lead to possible risk factors for food allergies. Low concentration of vitamin D is reported to increase the risk of peanut allergy, decrease the differentiation of pTregs, and activate Th2 polarization.

The microbiota hypothesis. The presence of particular bacterial strains, their metabolites, and some dietary substrates may promote the development of food allergies.

However, so far there is insufficient evidence to confirm or prove all these conceptual interpretations [2].

Food allergies are characterized by polymorphic clinical signs, which may manifest in any body system, particularly in such target organs as the gut, skin, unified airway, and genitourinary tract. They include swelling of the lips, tongue, or larynx, hives, skin rash and itching, bronchospasms, difficulty swallowing, feeling sick or vomiting, abdominal pain, or diarrhea, angioedema, etc. Swelling of the larynx may be life-threatening due to shortness of breath and even respiratory arrest.

Food allergies are reported to develop in different phenotypes such as classic, cross-reactive, aerosolized, and α-Gal syndrome (mammalian meat allergy), among which basic atopic sensitization due to IgE overproduction is predominant [90]. Besides phenotypes, food allergy endotypes, persistent, transient, local and systemic reactions, and drugs/exercise/alcohol-induced forms are described [90].

According to [91, 92], there are the following phenotype groups of food allergies:

1. IgE-mediated group (classically, of type I hypersensitivity by Gell and Coombs [93]), which includes acute urticaria and angioedema, allergic asthma, delayed food-induced anaphylaxis to mammalian meat, oral allergy syndrome, gastrointestinal allergic immediate reaction, and food anaphylaxis; this group is subdivided into (1) primary (with sensitization to Class 1 food allergens) and (ii) secondary food allergies (with hypersensitivity to Class 2 food allergens, for example, oral allergy syndrome);

2. Mixed group: atopic dermatitis and eosinophil-associated gastrointestinal inflammatory disease;

3. CD4+ T-cell-mediated group (classically, of type IV hypersensitivity by Gell and Coombs [93]) that includes celiac disease [41], food protein-induced enterocolitis syndrome (FPIES) [94], food protein-induced proctocolitis, and food protein-induced enteropathy.

In general, IgE-dependent food allergies are prevalent according to the classification.

It is fitting to highlight that phenotype is a recognizing feature of a disease, such as morphological, physiological, or biochemical property, or behavior, with no implication of a cell/molecular mechanism. Endotype represents a different physiological or pathological approach, which involves and uncovers cell and molecular mechanisms of a disease and response to therapy. Both phenotype and endotype are dependent on genotype and epigenetic modifications as well as environmental factors [2, 90, 95].

In the opinion of Chong et al. [86], most food allergy studies are devoted to either not persistent cases of food allergies or anaphylaxis. So far, such phenotypes as oral allergy syndrome (or pollen food allergy syndrome) [1, 7, 96], sporadic mild or moderate food allergies, and not truly life-threatening and really severe life-threatening anaphylaxis may be considered relatively studied [86]. Eosinophilic esophagitis [54] based on a high level of eosinophilic inflammation is a separate, strong genetically associated allergic disease [91]. Also, other rarer food allergy conditions than prevalent IgE disorders are outside of the scope of this chapter.

The cross-reaction if oral allergy syndrome occurs can be explained by the structural similarity of allergens, which may be found in both pollens and food. The list of cross-reactions is large and continuously expanding. Common examples are sensitization to birch, elm, and alder linked with food allergy to apple, peach, cherry, tomato, carrot, etc., and hypersensitivity to ragweed associated with a food allergy to watermelon, banana, zucchini, cucumber, etc. In addition, allergy to grass is associated with hypersensitivity to honey, orange, melon, etc. [6]. Chitinases are a group of allergens often found in plant food (wheat, rice, tomato, raspberry, grape, banana, coffee, etc.), latex (hevein), arthropods like house dust mites (HDM), and insects (silkworm). Accordingly, chitinases develop cross-reactivity syndrome and may even lead to anaphylaxis [97]. Most people can become tolerant of the cross-allergy if food products containing heat-labile allergens have been baked, cooked, and roasted.

There is currently no explanation for why life-threatening anaphylaxis occurs in only some atopic individuals among those who are allergic to food allergens [51, 98]. Genetic and epigenetic factors in food anaphylaxis are of high interest and are directly and indirectly involved in IgE-mediated food sensitization. Genetic background plays a significant role in the manifestation of most atopic diseases, whereas epigenetics matters greatly through three epigenetic mechanisms: DNA methylation, covalent posttranslational histone modifications, and micro-RNA-mediated gene silencing. Therefore, it may be essential for the interactions between various susceptibility genes, epigenetic modifications, immunologic processes, nerve impulses, and environmental factors [99]. However, explicit monogenic mutations linked with only anaphylaxis have not been found, but separate facts about some mutations causing anaphylaxis-like conditions and metabolic disturbances have continuously been accumulating [91]. It is likely that patients prone to more severe food allergies and also poorer outcomes in oral AIT have a specific phenotype [86], which is not yet confirmed by fundamental research findings.

In general, the series of prerequisites why life-threatening anaphylaxis occurs in only some individuals among those who are sensitized to food allergens is as follows [5]:

- polygeneous hereditary predisposition to atopy;
- individual hypersensitivity to selected allergens;
- dose and pathway of allergen entry specific for a patient;
- repeated penetration of the same allergen, which already caused anaphylaxis;

Criteria	Food anaphylaxis	Drug- or insect venom-induced anaphylaxis
Common manifestation age	Children	All ages
Prevalent signs and symptoms	Respiratory	Cardiovascular
Predominant route of allergen penetration	Oral, skin, or respiratory	Parenteral
Common onset time	Within 2 hours after exposure to allergen	Rapidly
Death cause	Respiratory arrest	Cardiac arrest
Mast cell tryptase as biomarker [100]	Moderate positive or negative	Positive

Table 3.
Peculiarities of food and nonfood-related anaphylaxis ([86], modified).

- acquired genetic alterations and epigenetic modifications promoting the weakness of the allergen tolerance maintenance system;

- peculiarities of forming memory T and B cells to food allergens [3].

Anaphylaxis in food allergies is observed more often than in drug- and insect venom-induced cases and shows some particular features important for differential diagnosis (see **Table 3**).

Food allergies frequently coexist with other atopic diseases, such as atopic dermatitis, allergic rhinitis, and allergic asthma. In comparison with children without food allergies, children sensitized to food allergens are two to four times more likely to suffer from asthma, particularly poorly controlled asthma [101]. Intake of snails in patients allergic to HDM can exacerbate the course of severe asthma, and airborne allergens such as wheat, fish, and seafood may result in so-called "food-induced asthma" [102]. Children co-sensitized to food and aero-allergens suffer from more severe clinical signs of allergic rhinitis [103].

However, a food allergy in isolation does not look like a typical atopic disease and it is rather not a chronic atopic disease but a series of discrete allergic episodes. That is because the gastrointestinal tract is a specific target organ unlike the other target organs being a zone allergen tolerance; therefore, food allergies may be a known exception to the rule conceived by evolution [5].

7. Diagnosis and management of food allergies

The diagnosis of a food allergy is very complex, requiring a detailed past medical history (or allergy anamnesis), physical examination, CRD [19, 104], BAT [22], SPT [24], and repeated visits to an allergist. Allergic skin tests, particularly SPT, occupy a central place in the diagnosis of food allergies. However, if a skin test is not suitable for revealing the food sensitization, a specific IgE determination is recommended [92]. An oral food challenge (or controlled food provocation test) may be administered, which an allergist conducts in the allergist's office taking into consideration the risk of an unpredictable severe allergic reaction like anaphylaxis. Nevertheless, the oral food challenge currently represents the "gold standard" diagnostic test due to the difficulty of food allergy diagnosis [105]. In relation to all diagnostic allergy tests, the main rule is that they must be used in combination, be guided by the medical history and be clinically relevant [92].

Treatment management of food allergies [106] consists in educating the patient about allergen avoidance, prescribing pharmacotherapy [92], biologics [106, 107], and AIT [108–111]. Urgently in anaphylaxis, an epinephrine auto-injector must be used. Once the diagnosis of food allergy is confirmed, strict elimination of the causative food allergen from the nutrition is absolutely necessary during lifespan; this allergen source can be replaced with another food product or, at least, if a causative allergen is heat-labile, be processed by baking, roasting, or boiling. Treatment of acute food reactions involves the prescription of epinephrine, antihistamines, glucocorticosteroids, and bronchodilators. Biologics can be applied as monotherapy or as adjuvant therapy to AIT.

AIT is a single method in IgE-mediated food allergies, which is disease-modified, well-documented, effective, and high-level medicine-based treatment option leading in allergen tolerance establishment [23, 92, 112]. In food allergies four routes of AIT were historically used: subcutaneous, sublingual, oral, and epicutaneous. Unfortunately, research into subcutaneous AIT in food allergies displayed severe systemic adverse effects, therefore many observations had been discontinued. Nevertheless, the subcutaneous route with peanut allergoid exhibited better tolerability [113]. Sublingual AIT displayed clinical efficacy and good tolerability but to a smaller extent than those in oral AIT, however, in a study with the use of standardized birch pollen extract better efficacy was described [114]. Epicutaneous AIT in patients with peanut allergies is currently undergoing a clinical trial.

Nowadays, research into the oral route of AIT in food allergies is actually at the cutting-edge. At the beginning of AIT (the up-dosing period) the daily oral administration of small but gradually increasing amounts of food allergen is conducted under medical supervision. The causative allergen is in-taken with food, and physical activity is avoided 2 hours after [115]. After completion of the up-dosing period, a daily maintenance dose may be in-taken at home. The oral route of AIT induces desensitization, irrespective of whether achievement of persistent tolerance is not yet evident. In the course of oral AIT, mild and moderate adverse reactions may be frequent, for example, mouth or throat itching and swelling, abdominal pain, but the risk of anaphylaxis and eosinophilic esophagitis remains. In 2020, Food and Drug Administration (FDA) approved the first licensed oral AIT product for peanut allergy—Palforzia® [116]. However, Palforzia® cannot be used in untreated or uncontrolled asthma and existing problems related to the esophagus and the gut. The European Academy of Allergy and Clinical Immunology (EAACI) prepared the guidelines on AIT for IgE-dependent food allergies. Trials have found substantial benefits for cow's milk, hen's egg, and peanut allergies, but a better adverse effect profile and high efficacy for oral AIT with cow's milk and hen's egg have not yet been confirmed. However, low-dose AIT may be useful in children with severe cow's milk allergy [117], but allergens has to be administered with caution to patients with a history of anaphylaxis [118]. AIT with food allergens should be exclusively performed in clinical centers with significant experience in such immunotherapy that patients should frequently visit during the up-dosing period. Patients must also make an informed decision about the therapy [119]. The dual-allergen exposure hypothesis is a precise reproduction of one of the mechanisms by which food allergies may develop; therefore, the hypothesis has been studied and discussed most extensively [119]. Furthermore, it is based on fundamental immune tolerance theory [120], which, if clinically experienced can be a good rationale for food allergy prevention using the approach of early introduction of food allergens in babies.

Prevention of food allergies by early introduction of food has been disputed. Some researchers suggest that the early introduction of peanut, cooked eggs, cow's milk, sesame, white fish, and wheat in exclusively breastfed infants at the age of 3 months with a hereditary risk of developing food allergies would reduce the prevalence of food allergy by the age 3 [6]. The idea of early introduction of allergenic food corresponds to the dual-allergen exposure hypothesis [89, 121], but, so far, it did not show clinical efficacy in relation to all those food allergens [88, 122].

Since food allergy patterns are different in distinct countries, for example, wheat allergy is prevalent in Japan and Thailand, whereas shellfish hypersensitivity is predominant in Singapore and the Philippines, the study of early introduction of potentially allergenic food has to be continued in children at high risk [123, 124]. In fact, the early introduction of food allergens during food intake is a natural induction of allergen tolerance, while AIT is an artificial medical approach.

Natural recovery from food sensitization is possible in infants depending on the allergen source, for example, cow's milk, hen's eggs, and wheat. Reverting a food allergy to allergen tolerance is the main purpose of AIT and is characterized by a loss of Th2 cells and an increase in Th1 cells, the simultaneous induction of blocking IgG antibodies, and suppression of inflammation's effector cell functions [23].

8. Oral tolerance

The logical completion of the chapter is a reference to oral tolerance, a state, which has to be recovered if a food allergy occurs. Simultaneously, oral tolerance enables the discussion of all questions related to food allergies and connected to food allergies as a challenge at present time.

This health condition is an organ-specific form of allergen tolerance, which is, in turn, a particular form of immune tolerance. However, there is not any separate oral tolerance since it exists in terms of combined allergen tolerance. In general, tolerance represents an antipode to active immune responses, which leads to the production of effector T cells and immunoglobulins participating in an "immune battle" against "non-self" or "former self". When an invader is defeated, the immune response has to complete the turning into tolerance. If tolerance does not develop, many types of pathology may manifest. Food allergies are a particular case because food proteins, glycoproteins, and lipoproteins are not dangerous invaders at all, and the immune response to them occurs by error. However, food allergies exist exhibiting a growing prevalence, and can become life-threatening, therefore, from an evolutionary viewpoint, oral tolerance maintenance has to be a solution to the challenge.

Oral tolerance must meet the following main criteria:

1. a potent allergen tolerance maintenance system in the gut,

2. balance in the intestinal microbiota with a significant amount of useful tolerogenic microbes, and.

3. integrity of the gastrointestinal barriers.

Oral tolerance depends on multiple factors, which can maintain or destabilize it under the daily penetration of food proteins, instability in the gut microbiota, changing signals from neuro molecules, and continuous trafficking of pro-inflammatory cells and molecules. The *dual-allergen exposure hypothesis* confirms a classical postulate of immune tolerance since the time of Burnet [121] that tolerance depends on age. If atopy predisposed babies before 3 months of age begin to consume peanuts this diet could decrease the risk of a peanut allergy after 12 months. In contrast, when such infants do not consume peanuts the likelihood of food allergy increases in the near future [6, 43]. Another important factor for oral tolerance breakdown is a high continuous dose of food allergens to which exposure may be available because of food intake and dietary preferences are daily and permanent.

In addition, impaired epithelial barrier integrity of the mouth predisposes a person to food allergies, in particular profilins-containing allergens, such as vegetables, fruits, seeds, and plant-based products [125]. Frequently disregarded mouth pathologies appear to present the prerequisites for food allergy manifestation confirming the existence of the oral route for rapid penetration of food allergens, which some researchers prefer to consider only as supplementary and even rare. Meanwhile, a healthy oral cavity is very significant in terms of food allergy prevention. Inflammatory processes in the gut result in increased epithelial permeability, facilitate food components to meet the submucosal immune cells and, under a deficiency of tolerogenic activity, trigger a Th2 pathway adaptive response or other IgE-independent pathogenetic mechanisms of food allergies [2, 23, 29, 88]. In sections 3 and 4, we described the high significance of the tolerogenic microbiota and ENIS in oral tolerance maintenance.

In the face of food allergies and inflammatory processes in the gut, evolution created the natural system of long-lasting oral tolerance maintenance enforced by the following components [5]:

- TDCs, including intestine-specific CD103+ TDC [4, 42];
- allergen-specific FoxP3 + pTreg cells [126, 127], as well as type 1 regulatory T (Tr1) cells and type 3 helper T (Th3) cells [128–130];
- regulatory B (Breg) cells [127, 128] and blocking antibodies;
- Peyer's patch and lamina propria M2 macrophages [4, 47];
- immunosuppressive cytokines: IL-10, transforming growth factor β (TGF-β), and IL-35 [5, 42, 43];
- pro-tolerogenic neurotransmitters and neuropeptides [5, 73, 79];
- tolerogenic microbiota [59–63].

Intestinal CD103 + DCs commonly endocyte food allergens penetrating through the epithelial barrier in readiness to promote Th2 pathway, however, metabolic products of tolerogenic microbiota, such as short-chain fatty acids and retinoid acid assign tolerogenic properties to these DCs turning them into CD103 + TDCs. TDC migrate into the mesenteric lymph nodes where they induce naïve T cells to mature into FoxP3 + pTreg cells using TGF-β and retinoid acid [4] and tolerize allergen-specific effector lymphocytes, making them anergic. Mature pTregs using expressed chemokine receptor CCR9 and integrin α4β7 arrive in the gut subepithelial region and along with TDC contribute to allergen tolerance to food allergens.

TDC and pTreg cells [42, 126, 131–133] play a general role in oral tolerance acting in a synergic manner to provide (1) the synthesis of IL-10, TGF-β, IL-35, and enzymes producing toxic for effector lymphocytes derivates like kynurenines; (2) expression of coinhibitory molecules, such as PD-1, CTLA-4, BTLA, and LAG-3 [134] known as antagonists of costimulatory molecules required for immune response forwarding; (3) competition with proliferative lymphocytes for the essential growth factor IL-2 [132]; (4) inhibition of Th1, Th2, Th17, and Th22 pathways [132] and many inflammatory cells like ILC2; (5) activation of follicular regulatory T (Tfr) cells [135], which downregulate Tfh cells. Subsets of pTregs are Tr1 and Th3 cells specialized for the mucosal barrier sites acting in a pTreg-like manner using the same mechanisms. Tr1 cells are known as $FoxP3^-$ IL-10-secreting Tregs [130], whereas Th3 cells are recognized as $FoxP3^-$ TGF-β-secreting Tregs [129]. In addition, there are pTreg subsets functionally directed to certain helper T cell subpopulations [129, 132] and memory pTregs [126, 127, 132].

B cells also generate a regulatory subset called Bregs. Breg cells contribute to oral tolerance secreting protolerogenic cytokines like IL-10, TGF-β, and IL-35, which upregulate IgG_4 production and downregulate IgE synthesis by plasma cells [136].

Peyer's patch and lamina propria M2 macrophages originate from circulating monocytes and exert tolerogenic properties by secretion of IL-10 and synergistically functioning along with pTregs [4].

IL-10 is the most potent immunosuppressive cytokine. In terms of the effects of TDC, pTregs, and other above-mentioned cells with tolerogenic properties, IL-10 inhibits the Th1 and Th2 pathways, expression of costimulatory molecules on allergen-presenting cells and lymphocytes, and activity of many inflammatory cells [42]. More or less, TGF-β and IL-35 display the analogous properties as IL-10.

GABA and serotonin are the most potent protolerogenic neurotransmitters in the ENIS with very rare exceptions, whereas neuropeptides CGRP and VIP can exhibit ambivalent effects depending on the microenvironment (see **Table 2** and **Figure 3** in Section 4). Nowadays, research into the influence of neuro molecules over oral tolerance is currently at the cutting-edge.

In the ENIS framework, the tolerogenic microbiota implements a unique role [61] in deterrence of the opportunistic bacteria growth and generation of metabolites and neuro molecules for TDCs and pTregs proliferation without which the gut and the whole body cannot exist since there are many other forms of gastrointestinal activity and gut-based vital functions.

In summary, oral tolerance to food and its loss occurs from a complicated interaction between the allergens in the food, the microbiota inhabiting the gut, intestinal epithelium integrity, immune and non-immune cells in the GALT, and protolerogenic neurotransmitters and neuropeptides found in the ENIS. If oral tolerance breaks down, the state may be recovered using the therapeutic approach called AIT with food allergens.

9. Conclusions

Food allergies are characterized by some routes of food allergen penetration and polymorphic clinical signs, which may manifest in anybody system, not only through the gut and in the gut. Normally, the intestine is a zone of tolerance in contrast with a place of immune responses to nutrients because evolution created the gastrointestinal tract as a container for food digestion, inhabitance of tolerogenic microbiota, and source of neuro molecules, hormones, and cytokines derived from the enteric neuroimmune system (ENIS).

The gut epithelium is a complex barrier membrane between the intestinal lumen and subepithelial region rich in cells and molecules of the ENIS. Single-cell RNA-sequencing, a transcriptomic technology, allowed to describe the novel composition of epitheliocytes and interepithelial cells, which were unknown in past [27, 28]. Nowadays, research on neuroimmune regulation of the gut has acquired a particular significance [76]. Nevertheless, food allergies caused by global changes on the planet and the new living environment for mankind are a violation of the rules conceived by evolution [5] and challenges for human civilization.

Allergen-specific immunotherapy (AIT) with food allergens can become an efficient approach for therapeutic management of this increasing pathology. Researchers have begun to describe the molecular structure of food allergens and have performed chip-based assays for many allergens. A study of the structure of culprit food allergens has allowed engineering synthetic and recombinant vaccines for AIT [1]. In addition, the idea of early introduction of allergenic food in infants, which corresponds to the dual-allergen exposure hypothesis [89, 121], is, in fact, another perspective approach for food allergy prevention [6, 123, 124].

Funding

This chapter received no external funding.

Conflict of interest

We confirm there are no conflicts of interest.

Author details

Vladimir Klimov*, Natalia Cherevko, Natalia Koshkarova and Andrew Klimov
Siberian State Medical University, Tomsk, Russia

*Address all correspondence to: klimov@mail.tomsknet.ru; vlklimov54@gmail.com

References

[1] Valenta R, Hochwallner H, Linhart B, Pahr S. Food allergies: The basics. Gastroenterology. 2015;**148**(6):1120-1131. DOI: 10.1053/j.gastro.2015.02.006

[2] Sicherer SH, Dampson HA. Food allergy: A review and update on epidemiology, pathogenesis, diagnosis, prevention, and management. The Journal of Allergy and Clinical Immunology. 2018;**141**(1):41-58. DOI: 10.1016/j.jaci.2017.11.003

[3] Koenig JFE, Bruton K, Phelps A, Grydziuszko E, Jimenez-Saiz R, Jordana M. Memory generation and re-activation in food allergy. ImmunoTargets and Therapy. 2021;**10**:171-184. DOI: 10.2147/ITT.S284823

[4] Liu EG, Yin X, Swaminathan A, Eisenbarth SC. Antigen-presenting cells in food tolerance and allergy. Frontiers in Immunology. 2021;**11**:616020. DOI: 10.3389/fimmu.2020.616020

[5] Klimov VV. Textbook of Allergen Tolerance. 1st ed. Cham: Springer; 2022. Forthcoming

[6] Waserman S, Beegin P, Watson W. IgE-mediated food allergy. Allergy, Asthma and Clinical Immunology. 2018;**14**(2):71-81. DOI: 10.1186/s13223-018-0284-3

[7] Jeon YH. Pollen-food allergy syndrome in children. Clinical and Experimental Pediatrics. 2020;**63**(12):463-468. DOI: 10.3345/cep.2019.00780

[8] Jeebhay MF, Moscato G, Bang BE, Folleti I, Lipinska-Ojrzanowska A, Lopata AL, et al. Food processing and occupational respiratory allergy—An EAACI position paper. Allergy. 2019;**74**:1852-1871. DOI: 10.1111/all.13807

[9] Pali-Schöll I, Verhoeckz K, Mafra I, Bavaro S, Mills ENC, Monaci L. Allergenic and novel food proteins: State of the art and challenges in the allergenicity assessment. Trends in Food Science and Technology. 2019;**84**:45-48. DOI: 10.1016/j.tifs.2018.03.007

[10] Fu L, Cherayil BJ, Shi H, Wang Y, Zhu Y. Allergenicity evaluation of food proteins. In: Food Allergy. Singapore: Springer; 2019. pp. 93-122. DOI: 10.1007/978-981-13-6928-5_5

[11] Hayes M. Chapter 14. Allergenicity of food proteins. In: Hayes M, editor. Novel Proteins for Food, Pharmaceuticals and Agriculture: Sources, Applications and Advances. Chichester: Wiley; 2018. pp. 269-280. DOI: 10.1002/9781119385332.ch14

[12] De Angelis E, Bavaro SL, Pilolli R, Monaci L. Food and nutritional analysis. Allergenic ingredients. In: Worsfold P, Townshend A, editors. Encyclopedia of Analytical Science. Amsterdam: Elsevier; 2019. pp. 349-373. DOI: 10.1016/B978-0-12-409547-2.13957-5

[13] Verhoeckx KCM, Vissers YM, Baumert JL, Faludi R, Feys M, Flanagan S, et al. Food processing and allergenicity. Food and Chemical Toxicology. 2015;**80**:223-240. DOI: 10.1016/j.fct.2015.03.005

[14] Francis OL, Wang KY, Kim EH, Moran TP. Common food allergens and cross-reactivity. Journal of Food Allergy. 2020;**2**(1):17-21. DOI: 10.2500/jfa.2020.2.200020

[15] Chan SK, Pomés A, Hilger C, Davies JM, Mueller G, Kuehn A, et al. Keeping allergen names clear and defined. Frontiers in Immunology. 2019;**10**:2600. DOI: 10.3389/fimmu.2019.02600

[16] Lowenstein H. Quantitative immunoelectrophoretic methods as a tool for the analysis and isolation of allergens. Progress Allergy. 1978;**25**:1-62. DOI: 10.1159/000401700

[17] Caraballo L, Valenta R, Acevedo N, Zakzuk J. Are the terms major and minor allergens useful for precision allergology? Frontiers in Immunology. 2021;**12**:651500. DOI: 10.3389/fimmu.2021.651500

[18] Breiteneder H, Diamant Z, Eiwegger T, Fokkens WJ, Traidl-Hoffmann C, Nadeau K, et al. Future research trends in understanding the mechanisms underlying allergic diseases for improved patient care. Allergy. 2019;**74**:2293-2311. DOI: 10.1111/all.13851

[19] Matricardi PM, Dramburg S, Potapova E, Skevaki C, Renz H. Molecular diagnosis for allergen immunotherapy. The Journal of Allergy and Clinical Immunology. 2019;**143**(3):831-843. DOI: 10.1016/j.jaci.2018.12.1021

[20] Van Hage M, Hamsten C, Valenta R. ImmunoCAP assays: Pros and cons in allergology. The Journal of Allergy and Clinical Immunology. 2017;**140**(4): 974-977. DOI: 10.1016/j.jaci.2017.05.008

[21] Di Fraia M, Arasi S, Castelli S, Dramburg S, Potapova E, Villalta D, et al. A new molecular multiplex IgE assay for the diagnosis of pollen allergy in Mediterranean countries: A validation study. Clinical and Experimental Allergy. 2019;**49**(3):341-349. DOI: 10.1111/cea.13264

[22] Santos AF, Lack G. Basophil activation test: Food challenge in a test tube or specialist research tool? Clinical and Translational Allergy. 2016;**6**:10. DOI: 10.1186/s13601-016-0098-7

[23] Schoos A-MM, Bullens D, Chawes BL, De Vlieger L, DunnGalvin A, Epstein MM, et al. Immunological outcomes of allergen-specific immunotherapy in food allergy. Frontiers in Immunology. 2020;**11**:568598. DOI: 10.3389/fimmu.2020.568598

[24] Heinzerling L, Mari A, Bergmann K-C, Bresciani M, Burbach G, Darsow U, et al. The skin prick test—European standards. Clinical and Translational Allergy. 2013;**3**(1):1-10. DOI: 10.1186/2045-7022-3-3

[25] Mansouri M, Rafiee E, Darougar S, Mesdaghi M, Chavoshzadeh Z. Is the atopy patch test reliable in the evaluation of food allergy-related atopic dermatitis? International Archives of Allergy and Immunology. 2018;**175**(1-2):85-90. DOI: 10.1159/000485126

[26] Larenas-Linnemann D, Luna-Pech JA, Mësges R. Debates in allergy medicine: Allergy skin testing cannot be replaced by molecular diagnosis in the near future. WAO Journal. 2017;**10**(32):1-7. DOI: 10.1186/s40413-017-0164-1

[27] Burclaff J, Bliton RJ, Breau KA, Ok MT, Gomez-Martinez I, Ranek JS, et al. A proximal-to-distal survey of healthy adult human small intestine and colon epithelium by single-cell transcriptomics. Cellular and Molecular Gastroenterology and Hepatology. 2022;**13**(5):1554-1589. DOI: 10.1016/j.jcmgh.2022.02.007

[28] Elmentaite R, Kumasaka N, Roberts K, Fleming A, Dann E, King HW, et al. Cells of the human

intestinal tract mapped across space and time. Nature. 2021;**597**:250-255. DOI: 10.1038/s41586-021-03852-1

[29] Ali A, Tan HY, Kaiko GE. Role of the intestinal epithelium and its interaction with the microbiota in food allergy. Frontiers in Immunology. 2020;**11**:604054. DOI: 10.3389/fimmu.2020.604054

[30] Newberry RD, Hogan SP. Intestinal epithelial cells in tolerance and allergy to dietary antigens. The Journal of Allergy and Clinical Immunology. 2021;**147**(1):45-48. DOI: 10.1016/j.jaci.2020.10.030

[31] Knoop KA, Newberry RD. Goblet cells: Multifaceted players in immunity at mucosal surfaces. Mucosal Immunology. 2018;**11**:1551-1557. DOI: 10.1038/s41385-018-0039-y

[32] Pali-Schöll I, Jensen-Jarolim E. The concept of allergen-associated molecular patterns (AAMP). Current Opinion in Immunology. 2016;**42**:113-118. DOI: 10.1016/j.coi.2016.08.004

[33] Jacquet A. Characterization of innate immune responses to house dust mite allergens: Pitfalls and limitations. Frontiers in Allergy. 2021;**2**:662378. DOI: 10.3389/falgy.2021.662378

[34] Allaire JM, Crowley SM, Law HT, Chang SY, Ko HJ, Vallance BA. The intestinal epithelium: Central coordinator of mucosal immunity. Trends in Immunology. 2018;**39**:677-696. DOI: 10.1016/j.it.2018.04.002

[35] Noah TK, Knoop KA, McDonald KG, Gustafsson JK, Waggoner L, Vanoni S, et al. IL-13-induced intestinal secretory epithelial cell antigen passages are required for IgE-mediated food-induced anaphylaxis. Journal of Allergy and Clinical Immunology. 2019;**144**:1058-1073.e3. DOI: 10.1016/j.jaci.2019.04.030

[36] Lueschow SR, McElroy SJ. The Paneth cell: The curator and defender of the immature small intestine. Frontiers in Immunology. 2020;**11**:587. DOI: 10.3389/fimmu.2020.00587

[37] Ting H-A, van Moltke J. The immune function of tuft cells at gut mucosal surfaces and beyond. Journal of Immunology. 2019;**202**:1321-1329. DOI: 10.4049/jimmunol.1801069

[38] Modasia A, Parker A, Jones E, Stentz R, Brion A, Goldson A, et al. Regulation of enteroendocrine cell networks by the major human gut symbiont Bacteroides thetaiotaomicron. Frontiers in Microbiology. 2020;**11**:575595. DOI: 10.3389/fmicb.2020.575595

[39] Walsh KT, Zemper AE. The enteric nervous system for epithelial researchers: Basic anatomy, techniques, and interactions with the epithelium. Cellular and Molecular Gastroenterology and Hepatology. 2019;**8**:369-378. DOI: 10.1016/j.jcmgh.2019.05.003

[40] Sun T, Nguyen A, Gommerman JL. Dendritic cell subsets in intestinal immunity and inflammation. Journal of Immunology. 2020;**204**:1075-1083. DOI: 10.4049/jimmunol.1900710

[41] Vitale S, Picascia S, Gianfrani C. The cross-talk between enterocytes and intraepithelial lymphocytes. Molecular and Cellular Pediatrics. 2016;**3**(1):20. DOI: 10.1186/s40348-016-0048-4

[42] Raker VK, Domogalla MP, Steinbrink K. Tolerogenic dendritic cells for regulatory T cell induction in man. Frontiers in Immunology. 2015;**6**:569. DOI: 10.3389/fimmu.2015.00569

[43] Tordesillas L, Berin MC, Sampson HA. Immunology of food allergy. Immunity. 2017;**47**:32-50. DOI: 10.1016/j.immuni.2017.07.004

[44] Collin M, Bigley V. Human dendritic cell subsets: An update. Immunology. 2018;**154**:3-20. DOI: 10.1111/imm.12888

[45] Zheng H, Zhang Y, Pan J, Liu N, Qin L, Liu M, et al. The role of type 2 innate lymphoid cells in allergic diseases. Frontiers in Immunology. 2021;**12**:586078. DOI: 10.3389/fimmu.2021.586078

[46] Peng Y, DeKruyff R, Fang S-B, Satitsuksanoa P, Zhang W, Ramsey N. Innate lymphoid cells in allergic diseases and intervention. Frontiers in Allergy. 2022; Forthcoming

[47] Chiaranunt P, Tai SL, Ngai L, Mortha A. Beyond immunity: Underappreciated functions of intestinal macrophages. Frontiers in Immunology. 2021;**12**:749708. DOI: 10.3389/fimmu.2021.749708

[48] Huber M, Cato ACB, Ainooson GK, Freichel M, Tsvilovskyy V, Jessberger R, et al. Regulation of the pleiotropic effects of tissue-resident mast cells. The Journal of Allergy and Clinical Immunology. 2019;**144**:S31-S45. DOI: 10.1016/j.jaci.2019.02.004

[49] Porebski G, Kwiecien K, Pawica M, Kwitniewski M. Mas-related G protein-coupled receptor-X2 (MRGPRX2) in drug hypersensitivity reactions. Frontiers in Immunology. 2018;**9**:3027. DOI: 10.3389/fimmu.2018.03027

[50] Varricchi G, Rossi FW, Galdiero MR, Granata F, Criscuolo G, Spadaro G, et al. Physiological roles of mast cells: Collegium Internationale Allergologicum Update. 2019. International Archives of Allergy and Immunology. 2019;**179**:247-261. DOI: 10.1159/000500088

[51] Wang Y-H. Developing food allergy: A potential immunologic pathway linking skin barrier to gut. F1000Research. 2016;**5**(F1000 Faculty Rev):2660. DOI: 10.12688/f1000research.9497.1

[52] Bochner BS. The eosinophil. Annals of Allergy, Asthma, & Immunology. 2018;**121**(2):150-155. DOI: 10.1016/j.anai.2018.02.031

[53] Celakovska J, Bukac J. Food hypersensitivity reactions and peripheral blood eosinophilia in patients suffering from atopic dermatitis. Food and Agricultural Immunology. 2017;**28**(1):35-43. DOI: 10.1080/09540105.2016.1202209

[54] Khan S, Guo X, Liu T, Iqbal M, Jiang K, Zhu L, et al. An update on eosinophilic esophagitis: Etiological factors, coexisting diseases, and complications. Digestion. 2021;**102**: 342-356. DOI: 10.1159/000508191

[55] Ramirez GA, Yacoub M-R, Ripa M, Mannina D, Gariddi A, Saporiti N, et al. Eosinophils from physiology to disease: A comprehensive review. BioMed Research International. 2018;**9095275**:1-28. DOI: 10.1155/2018/9095275

[56] Abbas M, Moussa M, Akel H. Type I hypersensitivity reaction. In: StatPearls. Treasure Island: StatPearls Publishing [Internet]; 2021. Available from: https://www.ncbi.nlm.nih.gov/books/NBK560561/

[57] Klose CSN, Veiga-Fernandes H. Neuroimmune interactions in peripheral tissues. European Journal of Immunology. 2021;**51**:1602-1614. DOI: 10.1002/eji.202048812

[58] Godinho-Silva C, Cardoso F, Veiga-Fernandes H. Neuro-immune cell units: A new paradigm in physiology. Annual Review of Immunology. 2019;**37**:19-46. DOI: 10.1146/annurev-immunol-042718-041812

[59] Palm NW, de Zoete MR, Flavell RA. Immune-microbiota interactions in health and disease. Clinical Immunology. 2015;**159**(2):122-127. DOI: 10.1016/j.clim.2015.05.014

[60] Lee KH, Song Y, Wu W, Yu K, Zhang G. The gut microbiota, environmental factors, and links to the development of food allergy. Clinical and Molecular Allergy. 2020;**18**:2. DOI: 10.1186/s12948-020-00120-x

[61] de Oliveira GLV, Cardoso CRB, Taneja V, Fasano A. Editorial: Intestinal dysbiosis in inflammatory diseases. Frontiers in Immunology. 2021;**12**:727485. DOI: 10.3389/fimmu.2021.727485

[62] Ortiz GG, Loera-Rodriguez LH, Cruz-Serrano JA, Torres Sanchez ED, Mora-Navarro MA, Delgado-Lara DLC, et al. Gut-brain axis: Role of microbiota in Parkinson's disease and multiple sclerosis. In: Artis AS, editor. Eat, Learn, Remember. London, UK: IntechOpen; 2018. pp. 11-30. DOI: 10.5772/intechopen.79493

[63] Savidge TC. Epigenetic regulation of enteric neurotransmission by gut bacteria. Frontiers in Cellular Neuroscience. 2016;**9**:503. DOI: 10.3389/fncel.2015.00503

[64] Shu S-A, Yuen AWT, Woo E, Chu K-H, Kwan H-S, Yang G-X, et al. Microbiota and food allergy. Clinical Reviews in Allergy and Immunology. 2019;**57**:83-97. DOI: 10.1007/s12016-018-8723-y

[65] Lo BC, Chen GY, Nunez G, Caruzo R. Gut microbiota and systemic immunity in health and disease. International Immunology. 2020;**33**(4):197-209. DOI: 10.1093/intimm/dxaa079

[66] Canani RB, Paparo L, Nocerino R, Di Scala C, Della Gatta G, Maddalena Y, et al. Gut microbiome as target for innovative strategies against food allergy. Frontiers in Immunology. 2019;**10**:191. DOI: 10.3389/fimmu.2019.00191

[67] Iweala OI, Nagler CR. The microbiome and food allergy. Annual Review of Immunology. 2019;**37**:377-403. DOI: 10.1146/annurev-immunol-042718-041621

[68] Mangalam AK, Ochoa-Reparaz JO. Editorial: The role of the gut microbiota in health and inflammatory diseases. Frontiers in Immunology. 2020;**11**:565305. DOI: 10.3389/fimmu.2020.565305

[69] Vitetta L, Vitetta G, Hall S. Immunological tolerance and function: Associations between intestinal bacteria, probiotics, prebiotics, and phages. Frontiers in Immunology. 2018;**9**:2240. DOI: 10.3389/fimmu.2018.02240

[70] Bryce PJ. Balancing tolerance or allergy to food proteins. Trends in Immunology. 2016;**37**(10):659-667. DOI: 10.1016/j.it.2016.08.008

[71] Voisin T, Bouvier A, Chiu IV. Neuro-immune interactions in allergic diseases: Novel targets for therapeutics. International Immunology. 2017;**29**(6):247-261. DOI: 10.1093/intimm/dxx040

[72] Hodo TW, de Aquino MTP, Shimamoto A, Shanker A. Critical neurotransmitters in the neuroimmune network. Frontiers in Immunology.

2020;**11**:1869. DOI: 10.3389/fimmu.2020.01869

[73] Chesné J, Cardoso V, Veiga-Fernandes H. Neuro-immune regulation of mucosal physiology. Mucosal Immunology. 2019;**12**:10-20. DOI: 10.1038/s41385-018-0063-y

[74] Mittal R, Debs LH, Patel AP, Nguyen D, Patel K, O'Connor G, et al. Neurotransmitters: The critical modulators regulating gut-brain axis. Journal of Cellular Physiology. 2017;**232**(9):2359-2372. DOI: 10.1002/jcp.25518

[75] Auteri M, Zizzo MG, Serio R. GABA and GABA receptors in the gastrointestinal tract: From motility to inflammation. Pharmacological Research. 2015;**93**:11-21. DOI: 10.1016/j.phrs.2014.12.001

[76] Jacobson A, Yang D, Vella M, Chiu IM. The intestinal neuro-immune axis: Crosstalk between neurons, immune cells, and microbes. Mucosal Immunology. 2021;**14**:555-565. DOI: 10.1038/s41385-020-00368-1

[77] Kerage D, Sloan EK, Mattarollo SR, McCombe PA. Interaction of neurotransmitters and neurochemicals with lymphocytes. Journal of Neuroimmunology. 2019;**332**:99-111. DOI: 10.1016/j.jneuroim.2019.04.006

[78] Kabata H, Artis D. Neuro-immune crosstalk and allergic inflammation. The Journal of Clinical Investigation. 2019;**129**(4):1475-1482. DOI: 10.1172/JCI124609

[79] Chen C-S, Barnoud C, Scheiermann C. Peripheral neurotransmitters in the immune system. Current Opinion in Physiology. 2021;**19**:73-79. DOI: 10.1016/j.cophys.2020.09.009

[80] Bosmans G, Bassi GS, Florens M, Gonzalez-Dominguez E, Matteoli G, Boeckxstaens GE. Cholinergic modulation of type 2 immune responses. Frontiers in Immunology. 2017;**8**:1873. DOI: 10.3389/fimmu.2017.01873

[81] Herr N, Bode C, Duerschmied D. The effects of serotonin in immune cells. Frontiers in Cardiovascular Medicine. 2017;**4**:48. DOI: 10.3389/fcvm.2017.00048

[82] Roumier A, Béchade C, Maroteaux L. Serotonin and the immune system. In: Pilowsky PM, editor. Serotonin. The Mediator That Spans Evolution. Amsterdam: Elsevier; 2019. pp. 181-196. DOI: 10.1016/B978-0-12-800050-2.00010-3

[83] Iwasaki M, Akiba Y, Kaunitz JD. Recent advances in vasoactive intestinal peptide physiology and pathophysiology: Focus on the gastrointestinal system. F1000Research. 2019;**8**:1629. DOI: 10.12688/f1000research.18039.1

[84] Kadowaki M, Yamamoto T, Hayashi S. Neuro-immune crosstalk and food allergy: Focus on enteric neurons and mucosal mast cells. Allergology International. 2022;**71**(3):278-287. DOI: 10.1016/j.alit.2022.03.004

[85] Micossé C, von Meyenn L, Steck O, Kipfer E, Adam C, Simillion C, et al. Human "TH9" cells are a subpopulation of PPAR-g+ TH2 cells. Science Immunology. 2019;**4**(31):eaat5943. DOI: 10.1126/sciimmunol.aat5943

[86] Chong KW, Ruiz-Garcia M, Patel N, Boyle RJ, Turner PJ. Reaction phenotypes in IgE-mediated food allergy and anaphylaxis. Annals of Allergy, Asthma & Immunology. 2020;**124**:473-478. DOI: 10.1016/j.anai.2019.12.023

[87] Komi DEA, Wohrl S, Bielory L. Mast cell biology at molecular level: A comprehensive review. Clinical Reviews in Allergy and Immunology. 2020;**58**(3):342-365. DOI: 10.1007/s12016-019-08769-2

[88] Calvani M, Anania C, Caffarelli C, Martelli A, Miraglia Del Giudice M, et al. Food allergy: An updated review on pathogenesis, diagnosis, prevention and management. Acta Biomedica. 2020;**15**:91. DOI: 10.23750/abm.v91i11-S.10316

[89] Sikorska-Szaflik H, Sozanska B. Primary prevention of food allergy—Environmental protection beyond diet. Nutrients. 2021;**13**(6):2025. DOI: 10.3390/nu13062025

[90] Baker MG, Sampson HA. Phenotypes and endotypes of food allergy: A path to better understanding the pathogenesis and prognosis of food allergy. Ann Allergy, Asthma and Immunology. 2018;**120**:245-253. DOI: 10.1016/j.anai.2018.01.027

[91] Azouz NP, Rothenberg ME. Mechanisms of gastrointestinal allergic disorders. The Journal of Clinical Investigation. 2019;**129**(4):1419-1430. DOI: 10.1172/JCI124604

[92] Worm M, Reese I, Ballmer B, Beyer K, Bischoff SC, Bohle B, et al. Update of the S2k guideline on the management of IgE-mediated food allergies. Allergologie Select. 2021;**5**:195-243. DOI: 10.5414/ALX02257E

[93] Coombs PR, Gell PG. Classification of allergic reactions responsible for clinical hypersensitivity and disease. In: Gell RR, editor. Clinical Aspects of Immunology, 1968. Oxford: Oxford University Press; 1968. pp. 575-596

[94] Maciag MC, Bartnikas LM, Sicherer SH, Herbert LJ, Young MC, Matney F, et al. A slice of FPIES (food protein-induced enterocolitis syndrome): Insights from 441 children with FPIES as provided by caregivers in the International FPIES Association. The Journal of Allergy and Clinical Immunology. In Practice. 2020;**8**(5):1702-1709. DOI: 10.1016/j.jaip.2020.01.030

[95] Bellanti JA. Phenotypic classification of asthma based on a new Type 2-high and Type 2-low endotypic classification: It all began with Rackemann. J Prec Resp Med. 2020;**3**(1):9-20. DOI: 10.2500/jprm.2020.3.200001

[96] Carlson G, Coop C. Pollen food allergy syndrome (PFAS): A review of current available literature. Annals of Allergy, Asthma & Immunology. 2019;**123**:359-365. DOI: 10.1016/j.anai.2019.07.022

[97] Leoni C, Volpicella M, Dileo MCD, Gattulli BAR, Ceci LR. Chitinases as food allergens. Molecules. 2019;**24**(11):2087. DOI: 10.3390/molecules24112087

[98] Alcocer MJC, Ares SC, Lopez-Calleja. Recent advances in food allergy. Brazilian Journal of Food Technology. 2016;**19**:e2016047. DOI: 10.1590/1981-6723.4716

[99] Bellanti JA, Settipane RA. Genetics, epigenetics, and allergic disease: A gun loaded by genetics and a trigger pulled by epigenetics. Allergy and Asthma Proceedings. 2019;**40**(2):73-75. DOI: 10.2500/aap.2019.40.4206

[100] Beck SC, Wilding T, Buka RJ, Baretto RL, Huissoon AP, Krishna MT. Biomarkers in human anaphylaxis: A critical appraisal of current evidence and perspectives. Frontiers in Immunology. 2019;**10**:494. DOI: 10.3389/fimmu.2019.00494

[101] Chan A, Yu JE. Food allergy and asthma. Journal of Food Allergy. 2020;**2**(1):44-47. DOI: 10.2500/jfa.2020.2.200003

[102] Emons JAM, van Wijk GR. Food allergy and asthma: Is there a link? Current Treatment Options in Allergy. 2018;**5**:436-444. DOI: 10.1007/s40521-018-0185-1

[103] Wang Y-H, Lue K-H. Association between sensitized to food allergens and childhood allergic respiratory diseases in Taiwan. Journal of Microbiology, Immunology and Infection. 2020;**53**(5):812-820. DOI: 10.1016/j.jmii.2019.01.005

[104] Eiwegger T, Hung L, San Diego KE, O'Mahony L, Upton J. Recent developments and highlights in food allergy. Allergy. 2019;**74**(12):2355-2367. DOI: 10.1111/all.14082

[105] Foong R-X, Dantzer JA, Wood RA, Santos AF. Improving diagnostic accuracy in food allergy. The Journal of Allergy and Clinical Immunology. In Practice. 2021;**9**(1):71-80. DOI: 10.1016/j.jaip.2020.09.037

[106] Tontini C, Bulfone-Paus S. Novel approaches in the inhibition of IgE-induced mast cell reactivity in food allergy. Frontiers in Immunology. 2021;**12**:613461. DOI: 10.3389/fimmu.2021.613461

[107] Chen M, Zhang W, Lee L, Saxena J, Sindher S, Chinthrajah RS, et al. Biologic therapy for food allergy. Journal of Food Allergy. 2020;**2**(1):86-90. DOI: 10.2500/jfa.2020.2.200004

[108] Głobińska A, Boonpiyathad T, Satitsuksanoa P, Kleuskens M, van der Veen W, Sokolowska M, et al. Mechanisms of allergen-specific immunotherapy. Diverse mechanisms of immune tolerance to allergens. Annals of Allergy, Asthma, & Immunology. 2018;**121**:306-312. DOI: 10.1016/j.anai.2018.06.026

[109] Mäntylä J, Thomander T, Hakulinen A, Kukkonen K, Palosuo K, Voutilainen H, et al. The effect of oral immunotherapy treatment in severe IgE mediated milk, peanut, and egg allergy in adults. Immunity, Inflammation and Disease. 2018;**6**(2):307-311. DOI: 10.1002/iid3.218

[110] Nagakura K-I, Sato S, Yanagida N, Nishino M, Asaumi T, Ogura K, et al. Oral immunotherapy in Japanese children with anaphylactic peanut allergy. International Archives of Allergy and Immunology. 2018;**175**(3):181-188. DOI: 10.1159/000486310

[111] Sampath V, Nadeau KC. Newly identified T cell subsets in mechanistic studies of food immunotherapy. Journal of Clinical Investigation. 2019;**129**(4):1431-1440. DOI: 10.1172/JCI124605

[112] Fuhrmann V, Huang H-J, Akarsu A, Shilovskiy I, Elisyutina O, Khaitov M, et al. From allergen molecules to molecular immunotherapy of nut allergy: A hard nut to crack. Frontiers in Immunology. 2021;**12**:742732. DOI: 10.3389/fimmu.2021.742732

[113] Bindslev-Jensen C, de Kam P-J, van Twuojver E, Boot D, El Galta R, Mose AP, et al. SCIT-treatment with a chemically modified, aluminum hydroxide adsorbed peanut extract (HAL-MPE1) was generally safe and well tolerated and showed immunological changes in peanut allergic patients. The Journal of Allergy and Clinical Immunology. 2017;**139**(2):AB191. DOI: 10.1016/j.jaci.2016.12.623

[114] Till SJ, Stage BS, Skypala I, Biedermann T. Potential treatment effect of the SQ tree SLIT-tablet on pollen food syndrome caused by apple. Allergy. 2020;**75**(8):2059-2061. DOI: 10.1111/all.14242

[115] Feuille E, Nowak-Wegrzyn A. Allergen-specific immunotherapies for food allergy. Allergy, Asthma & Immunology Research. 2018;**10**(3):189-206. DOI: 10.4168/aair.2018.10.3.189

[116] Sood AK, Scurlock AM. Food allergy oral immunotherapy. Journal of Food Allergy. 2020;**2**(1):75-80. DOI: 10.2500/jfa.2020.2.200005

[117] Miura Y, Nagakura KI, Sato S, Yanagida N, Ebisawa M. Precision medicine for cow's milk immunotherapy in clinical practice. Current Opinion in Allergy and Clinical Immunology. 2021;**21**(4):378-385. DOI: 10.1097/ACI.0000000000000756

[118] Demir E, Günaydın NC, Gülen F, Tanaç R. Oral immunotherapy for cow's milk allergy: Five years' experience. Balkan Medical Journal. 2020;**37**:316-323. DOI: 10.4274/balkanmedj.galenos.2020.2020.1.140

[119] Pajno GB, Fernandez-Rivas M, Arasi S, Roberts G, Akdis CA, Alvaro-Lozano M, et al. EAACI Guidelines on allergen immunotherapy: IgE-mediated food allergy. Allergy. 2018;**73**(4):799-814. DOI: 10.1111/all.13319

[120] Burnet FM. Immunological Recognition of Self: Nobel Lecture. Nobel Foundation; 1960. Archived from the original on 15 December 2010

[121] Du Toit G, Sampson HA, Plaut M, Burks AW, Akdis CA, Lack G. Food allergy: Update on prevention and tolerance. The Journal of Allergy and Clinical Immunology. 2018;**141**(1):30-40. DOI: 10.1016/j.jaci.2017.11.010

[122] Leonard SA. Food allergy prevention, including early food introduction. Journal of Food Allergy. 2020;**2**(1):69-74. DOI: 10.2500/jfa.2020.2.200007

[123] Tham EH, Shek LP-C, Van Bever HPS, Vichyanond P, Ebisawa M, Wong GWK, et al. Early introduction of allergenic foods for the prevention of food allergy from an Asian perspective—An Asia Pacific Association of Pediatric Allergy, Respirology & Immunology (APAPARI) consensus statement. Pediatric Allergy and Immunology. 2018;**29**(1):18-27. DOI: 10.1111/pai.12820

[124] Chan ES, Abrams EM, Hildebrand KJ, Watson W. Early introduction of foods to prevent food allergy. Allergy, Asthma and Clinical Immunology. 2018;**14**(57):93-101. DOI: 10.1186/s13223-018-0286-1

[125] RosaceD,Gomez-CasadoC,FernandezP, Perez-Gordo M, Dominguez MD, Vega A, et al. Profilin-mediated food-induced allergic reactions are associated with oral epithelial remodeling. Journal of Allergy and Clinical Immunology. 2019;**143**(2):681-690.E1. DOI: 10.1016/j.jaci.2018.03.013

[126] Shevyrev D, Tereshchenko V. Treg heterogeneity, function, and homeostasis. Frontiers in Immunology. 2020;**10**:3100. DOI: 10.3389/fimmu.2019.03100

[127] Motos TR, Hirakawa M, Alho AC, Neleman L, Graca L, Ritz J. Maturation and phenotypic heterogeneity of human CD4+ regulatory T cells from birth to adulthood and after allogeneic stem cell transplantation. Frontiers in Immunology. 2021;**11**:570550. DOI: 10.3389/fimmu.2020.570550

[128] Abdel-Gadir A, Massoud AH, Chatila TA. Antigen-specific Treg cells in immunological tolerance: Implications for allergic diseases. F1000Research. 2018;**7**:1-13. DOI: 10.12688/f1000research.12650

[129] Calzada D, Baos S, Cremades-Jimeno L, Cardaba B. Immunological mechanisms in allergic diseases and allergen tolerance: The role of Treg cells. Hindawi. Journal of Immunology Research. 2018;**6012053**:1-10. DOI: 10.1155/2018/6012053

[130] Roncarolo MG, Gregpri S, Bacchetta R, Battaglia M, Gagliani N. The biology of T regulatory type 1 cells and their therapeutic application in immune-mediated diseases. Immunity. 2018;**49**(6):1004-1019. DOI: 10.1016/j.immuni.2018.12.001

[131] Abebe EC, Dejenie TA, Ayele TM, Baye ND, Teshome AA, Muche ZT. The role of regulatory B cells in health and diseases: A systemic review. Journal of Inflammation Research. 2021;**14**:75-84. DOI: 10.2147/JIR.S286426

[132] Kupriyanov SV, Sinitsky AI, Dolgushin II. Multiple subsets of regulatory T-cells. Bulletin of Siberian Medicine. 2020;**19**(3):144-155. DOI:10.20538/1682-0363-2020-3-144-155

[133] Kim KS, Hong S-W, Han D, Yi J, Jung J, Yang B-G, et al. Dietary antigens limit mucosal immunity by inducing regulatory T cells in the small intestine. Science. 2016;**351**(6275):858-863. DOI: 10.1126/science.aac5560

[134] Rosscopf S, Jahn-Schmid B, Schmetter KG, Zlabinger GJ, Steinberger P. PD-1 has a unique capacity to inhibit allergen-specific human CD4+ T cell responses. Scientific Reports. 2018;**8**:13543. DOI: 10.1038/s41598-018-31757-z

[135] Lu Y, Craft J. T follicular regulatory cells: Choreographers of productive germinal center responses. Frontiers in Immunology. 2021;**12**:679909. DOI: 10.3389/fimmu.2021.679909

[136] Satitsuksanoa P, Daanje M, Akdis M, Boyd SD, van de Veen W. Biology and dynamics of B cells in the context of IgE-mediated food allergy. Allergy. 2020;**76**(6):1707-1717. DOI: 10.1111/all.14684

Chapter 5

Anaphylaxis in Infants

Natalia Esakova, Alexander Nikolaevich Pampura, Nazifa Dustbabaeva and Venera Baybekova

Abstract

Anaphylaxis is an extremely dangerous systemic hypersensitivity reaction that develops rapidly and can be fatal. Infants make up the most difficult group of patients with anaphylaxis, given the first episode of reaction occurring at an early age, there are age-related difficulties in interpreting complaints, unpredictability of clinical symptoms, prolonged process of diagnosis, and prescribing the appropriate treatment. These factors determine the risk of fatal outcomes, even in case of nearly healthy infants. For this group of patients, such problems as lack of available diagnostic tests, limited standard doses of epinephrine autoinjectors, the absence of predictors of occurrence, and severity of systemic allergic reactions are still relevant. This chapter presents the available information on the prevalence of anaphylaxis, the most common triggers, diagnosis, clinical symptoms, severity, and treatment in infants.

Keywords: anaphylaxis, anaphylactic reaction, trigger, allergen, children, food allergy, infants, molecular diagnostics, specific IgE, tryptase

1. Introduction

Anaphylaxis is an extremely dangerous systemic hypersensitivity reaction that develops rapidly and can be fatal [1]. More than 120 years have passed since the phenomenon of anaphylaxis was first described, but there are still numerous difficulties and questions related to the management of patients with this diagnosis. Physicians' attention to the problem of anaphylaxis has revived over the last 20–30 years, due to the increased prevalence of systemic reactions to various triggers (food allergens, medications, latex, physical exercise, etc.). Infants make up the most difficult group of patients with anaphylaxis, given the first episode of reaction occurring at an early age, there are age-related difficulties in interpreting complaints, unpredictability of clinical symptoms, prolonged process of diagnosis, and prescribing the appropriate treatment. These factors determine the risk of fatal outcomes, even in the case of nearly healthy infants. For this group of patients, such problems as lack of available diagnostic tests, limited standard doses of epinephrine (adrenaline) autoinjectors, the absence of predictors of occurrence, and severity of systemic allergic reactions are still relevant. This chapter presents the available information on prevalence of anaphylaxis, the most common triggers, diagnosis, clinical symptoms, severity, and treatment in infants.

2. Prevalence

Data on prevalence and incidence of anaphylaxis in infants are limited, and the younger the child, the less reliable information is available regarding the problem, but anaphylaxis occurs even in two-week-old infants [2–4]. Results of the epidemiological studies are variable, largely due to dissimilar methodologies; for example, analysis of referrals to allergy clinics or emergency departments will differ from the evaluation of the international anaphylaxis registry database or medical records review (epinephrine auto-injector prescription, epicrisis, and ICD code) or general survey of respondents. There are some features of the definitions used in various clinical and epidemiological studies in infants (0–36 months). The term "infants" is usually used for children during the first 2 years of life; in some studies, "infants" refer to children under the first 12 months of life (which is additionally reported); "toddlers" refer to children between 12 and 36 months of life; some researchers randomly select age periods (e.g., from 0 to 4 years).

According to numerous studies that analyzed medical documentation databases, the incidence of anaphylaxis in infants during the first 4 years of life was 3–4 times higher than in other age groups. In the city of Alcorcon (Spain), the peak incidence of anaphylaxis was found in children under 4 years old and amounted to 313.58 per 100,000 person-year between 2004 and 2005 [5]. The figures were three times higher than in older age groups. In Australia, there were reports about an increase in hospitalizations due to anaphylaxis from 4.1 to 19.7 per 100,000 person-year in children under 4 years old [6].

A number of studies report that anaphylaxis in infants ranges from 25% to 34% of all pediatric anaphylaxis cases, and the incidence is slightly higher in boys (56–69%) than in girls [7–11]. According to Huang et al. [12], the share of patients <1 year of life was 3.1% out of 192 children with anaphylaxis admitted to emergency department. According to our research conducted in Russia at the pediatric allergy department, more than half of patients (58%) with food-induced anaphylaxis had their first reaction episode between the age of 8 months and 2 years [13].

In recent years, there has been an increase in the prevalence of the disease in infants, especially food-induced anaphylaxis. Motosue et al. [14] reported a 129% increase in the number of admissions to emergency departments due to anaphylactic reactions in infants during the first 5 years of life between 2005 and 2014. In the state of Illinois (USA), there was a 29% annual increase in the number of referrals and admissions to intensive care units due to food-induced anaphylaxis in infants aged 0–4 years in 2008–2012 [15]. For instance, the incidence of food-induced anaphylaxis in this age group totaled 11.9 cases per 100,000 person-year in 2008 and increased to 30.5 cases per 100,000 person-year in 2012.

The foregoing data demonstrate the vulnerability of infants to increasing prevalence and risk of anaphylaxis. It is of paramount importance to consider that most of the data are underreported and cannot fully reflect the real epidemiological pattern, since many episodes of anaphylactic reactions in infants occur for the first time and some of them are overlooked.

3. Triggers

Food is the main trigger of anaphylaxis in infants. In older children, food-induced allergy causes at least 50% of all anaphylactic reactions, and in younger patients, it is up to 70–90% [7, 16, 17]. According to the study conducted in New Zealand, the retrospective analysis of 10-year medical records of patients with ICD-9 code T78.0 (anaphylactic shock due to adverse food reaction) and T78.2 (anaphylactic shock unspecified) showed that incidence of food-induced anaphylaxis in patients under the age of 2 made up 50.5 per 100,000 person-year and significantly exceeded its rate in the total group of children (16.2 per 100,000 person-year) [18]. Colleagues in Singapore also demonstrated that the highest percentage of food-induced anaphylaxis cases occurs in infants under 2 years old (up to 90%), and the rate drops to 73% in children aged 2–11 [19].

Country	Authors	Study type	Number (N)	Age	Triggers		
					First place	Second place	Third place
Russia	Esakova et al., 2014 [13]	Retrospective analysis of medical records in tertiary hospital	N=46	0–2 years	Cow's milk (56,5%)	Hen's egg (15,2%)	Fish or/and seafood (13,1%)
China	Jiang et al., 2021 [17]	Retrospective analysis of medical records in tertiary hospital	N=134	0–2 years	Cow's milk (32,9%)	Hen's egg (21,4%)	Wheat (20,7%)
Korea	Jeon et al., 2019 [7]	Retrospective analysis of medical records in 23 secondary or tertiary hospitals	N=338	0–2 years	Cow's milk (43,8%)	Hen's egg (21,9%)	Walnut (8,3%)
France	Pouessel et al., 2020 [20]	Retrospective analysis of cases recorded by the allergy vigilance network	N=61	≤12 months	Cow's milk (59%)	Hen's egg (20%)	Wheat (7%)
USA	Rudders et al., 2011 [8]	Retrospective analysis of medical records in ED	N=61	0–2 years	Cow's milk (40%)	Peanut (31%)	Hen's egg (31%)
USA	Ko et al., 2020 [21]	Retrospective analysis of medical records in ED	N=448	≤12 months	Hen's egg (34%)	Peanut (22%)	Cow's milk (16%)
Turkey	Topal et al., 2017 [13]	Retrospective analysis of medical records in ED	N=23	≤12 months	Cow's milk (61%)	Hen's egg (21%)	Walnut (9%)
Turkey	Kahveci et al., 2020 [22]	Retrospective analysis of medical records in hospital	N=160	≤12 months	Cow's milk (51,4%)	Tree nuts (16,6%)	Hen's egg (15,4%)
Australia	Andrew et al., 2018 [23]	Retrospective analysis of medical records in EMS	N=127	≤12 months	Hen's egg (37,9%)	Tree nuts (31%)	Cow's milk (30,9%)
Spain	Alvarez-Perea et al., 2018 [24]	Retrospective analysis of medical records in ED	N=127	≤12 months	Cow's milk (67%)	Hen's egg (22%)	Fruits or fish (6%)

Table 1.
The most significant triggers of food anaphylaxis in infants.

Virtually any food can cause anaphylaxis in infants, but the most significant triggers in patients during the first years of life are cow's milk and hen's egg (**Table 1**). According to our data obtained in Russia, cow's milk (56.5%) and hen's egg (15.2%) were the most common allergens to cause food-induced anaphylaxis in infants <2 years of age [13]. It distinguishes them from older children because in this age group, tree nuts (29.4%), fish/seafood (26.5%), and fruit (23.5%) are the dominant triggers. Similar results are seen in studies from other countries. In the comparative study conducted in China, food allergens, such as cow's milk (32.9%), eggs (21.4%), and wheat (20.7%), were the most common triggers of anaphylaxis in infants <2 years of age, whereas in preschool (3–6 years) and school-aged children (7–12 years), fruits and vegetables (31.6% and 35.9%, respectively) were the major allergens [17]. In France, cow's milk (59%), hen's egg (20%), wheat (7%), and peanuts (3%) are the most frequent causes of anaphylaxis in infants <1 year of age [20]. According to Rudders et al. [8], cow's milk, peanuts, and hen's egg are the main triggers of anaphylactic reactions in infants <2 years of age in the United States, which is consistent with findings from another American study based on retrospective analysis of intensive care units' data covering the period between 2016 and 2018 [21]. Colleagues in Turkey also report that above 50% of food anaphylaxis cases in infants <1 year of age are associated with the consumption of cow's milk [11, 22]. In Australia, the most common trigger of anaphylaxis is hen's egg (39%) [23], in Spain, unlike in most countries, the top three allergens, along with cow's milk and eggs, include fruit and fish (9%) [24].

Sensitization to some allergens can occur at an early age when they are passed to a child in breast milk. So, anaphylaxis can occur both during breastfeeding (less common) and when the product is first consumed [25, 26]. Two cases of anaphylaxis in the form of urticaria, vomiting, cough, and wheeze have been described in exclusively breastfed infants during the first year of life and took place after the consumption of fish by the mother [26, 27]. Specific IgE to several types of fish was detected during the pediatric examination. In 1988, Lifschitz et al. [28] described a one-month-old patient with an anaphylactic reaction after consuming breast milk, which had been collected earlier before the child was found to be hypersensitive to cow's milk proteins; at that time, the mother was not following a dairy-free diet. In infants, anaphylactic reactions to various formulas, partially highly hydrolyzed, are possible [29]. Anaphylaxis can be induced by a high-hydrolysis formula not only in infants <1 year of age, a case of anaphylaxis after 3 years of milk elimination in a 5-year-old child during a provocation test with high-hydrolysis formula, sIgE level to cow's milk was 37.1 UA/mL (ImmunoCAP, Sweden) [30]. Cases of anaphylaxis after the first use of partial hydrolysate formula have been described in children who were previously exclusively breastfed with the exclusion of cow's milk protein by the mother [31].

Typically, cow's milk is the first foreign protein introduced into a child's diet, so it is one of the most frequent triggers of food anaphylaxis in infants. Pouessel et al. [20] reported that in 28 (46%) of 61 cases of anaphylaxis caused by cow's milk, the first episode of anaphylactic reaction was noted when this allergen was first consumed after cessation of breastfeeding. There are reports of anaphylaxis in infants with cow's milk allergy after the first consumption of goat's milk and soy-based formula [32]. Moreover, anaphylactic reactions in infants are possible even to less traditionally accepted products for this age: rare fruits and vegetables [33], seeds (pumpkin, sesame, and mustard) [34], different types of meat (e.g., caribou, whale) [35], bee products [36], etc.

One of the most difficult and unpredictable situations is anaphylaxis to hidden allergens, which sometimes are not mentioned in the product composition. Zurzolo et al. [37] conducted a survey involving 198 respondents with food allergies, who retrospectively evaluated the development of anaphylaxis after consuming packaged food that did not contain the allergen in question. The share of such anaphylactic reactions amounted to 7%. Sometimes parents themselves do not properly read the labels, which leads to repeated episodes of anaphylaxis. For example, there was a case at our clinic, when a girl suffering from food allergy since an early age had an episode of anaphylaxis after the first consumption of peanut sticks at the age of 1.5. As for clinical symptoms, pronounced swelling of the neck, breathing difficulties, sweating, pallor, cyanosis, and repeated vomiting were noted. After the first episode of anaphylaxis, the child's parents tried to avoid food that might contain peanuts. But despite all efforts, 6 months later the child had another episode of anaphylactic reaction after eating bread, which contained trace amounts of peanuts, but the parents did not consider that. Such cases are far from isolated.

We should not forget the possibility of accidental non-oral contact of the child with the causative product. For example, inhalation of aerosolized food particles during cooking and skin contact with allergens. According to our observation, the rate of patients with anaphylactic reactions caused by skin contact or inhalation of allergen amounts to 16.4% [38]. The predominant triggers of anaphylaxis caused by skin contact are fish/seafood allergens (46%) and cow's milk (33%), and the most common triggers of anaphylaxis caused by inhalation are fish/seafood allergens (89%).

Anaphylactic reactions to drugs occur in a small percentage of cases in infants. The most common triggers of drug-induced anaphylaxis in children are antibacterial drugs, as per Xing et al. Ref. [39] analysis of 91 cases of drug-induced anaphylaxis in children showed that the share of reactions to antibiotics amounted to 53%. Topal et al. [11] described one patient with anaphylaxis to antibacterial drug in a group of children under one year of age. Nonsteroidal anti-inflammatory drugs are in second place in terms of incidence of anaphylaxis induction. Gabrielli et al. [40] showed that antibacterial drugs triggered 37.3% of drug-induced anaphylaxis in children (mean age 3.8 years old), while nonsteroidal anti-inflammatory drugs caused 21.6% of cases.

Various medications contain residual amounts of a food allergen and can cause anaphylaxis in infants. There is a report of an 11-month-old infant with atopic dermatitis and allergy to cow's milk proteins who had anaphylaxis episode 15 minutes after consuming bacilor (Lyocentre Laboratories, Aurillac, France) containing Lactobacillus rhamnosus [41]. Prick test with bacilor was positive.

Vaccination poses a threat of anaphylaxis in infants. Most vaccinations occur in the first two years of life, so there is no anamnestic data regarding tolerability and risk of adverse reactions. A population-based study reported an anaphylaxis rate of 1.31 cases per 100,000,000 doses for all age groups [42]. Vaccines contain not only immunogenic determinants but also trace amounts of various components that may be allergens. Therefore, sensitization, which can induce anaphylaxis by vaccination, may develop before the use of the vaccine or during the first and subsequent injections. The most significant inducers of anaphylaxis include hen's egg allergens, antimicrobial agents, and gelatin. For example, hen's egg protein is present in significant amounts (μg/ml) in yellow fever, influenza, varicella, rabies, measles, and mumps vaccines, and this amount may be sufficient to develop anaphylactic reactions in patients with anaphylaxis to hen's eggs [43]. Antimicrobial agents, neomycin, streptomycin, kanamycin, and polymyxin B may be present in trace amounts in live virus vaccines, so patients with a history of anaphylactic reaction to these antibacterial agents should not receive vaccines containing these components [44]. As a stabilizer, gelatin is contained in high concentrations in the yellow fever vaccine (up to 72 mg/0.5 ml dose) and in some influenza vaccines (up to 250 mg/0.5 ml dose). Therefore, these vaccines may provoke anaphylaxis in patients highly sensitive to this component [45].

It is important that the presence of allergic diseases in the history of an infant is not necessarily a prerequisite for anaphylaxis. According to Pouessel et al. [20], 89% of children with food anaphylaxis in the first year of life had no previous food allergy; according to our observation, the proportion of such patients is up to 25% [13]. Among the cofactors that increase the risk of anaphylaxis in infants, Pouessel et al. [20] identified intake of proton pump inhibitor (esomeprazole) and acute respiratory infection at the time of anaphylactic reaction occurrence.

4. Clinical symptoms and diagnosis

4.1 Clinical criteria for diagnosis

In most cases, anaphylaxis in infants is typical and develops within a few seconds-minutes, usually within 2 hours after contact with the allergen, but regression of symptoms may develop gradually. Biphasic and protracted anaphylaxis are extremely rare in infants. The proportion of biphasic anaphylaxis is reported to be about 3–5% in infants with anaphylaxis <2 years of age [7]. There are isolated reports of biphasic anaphylaxis in infants. Lee et al. [46] described this form of anaphylaxis in two children aged 1 and 2 years. Pouessel et al. [20] described a case of the biphasic anaphylactic reaction of a 9-month-old child after consumption of a hen's egg; initially, there were symptoms in the form of vomiting, abdominal pain, and diffuse skin rash, which disappeared without any therapy, but 4 hours later the symptoms resumed and required epinephrine injection. Protracted anaphylaxis in infants is extremely rare. In our clinical practice, we observed an 8-month-old child with respiratory failure, angioedema, and generalized urticaria after the first consumption of three pine nuts. The child had repeated injections of epinephrine and artificial ventilation for 3 days.

To diagnose anaphylaxis, regardless of patient age, the 2005 clinical criteria of the Second National Institute of Allergy and Infectious Disease/Food Allergy and

Criteria	Characterization of symptoms [NIAID/FAAN, 2005]	Characterization of symptoms [WAOAG, 2020]
1	Acute onset of an illness (minutes to several hours) with involvement of the skin, mucosal tissue, or both (e.g., generalized hives, pruritus or flushing, swollen lips-tongue-uvula) And at least one of the following: a. Respiratory compromise (e.g., dyspnea, wheeze-bronchospasm, stridor, reduced PEF, hypoxemia); b. Reduced BP or associated symptoms of end-organ dysfunction (e.g., hypotonia [collapse], syncope, incontinence).	Acute onset of an illness (minutes to several hours) with simultaneous involvement of the skin, mucosal tissue, or both (e.g., generalized hives, pruritus or flushing, swollen lips-tongue-uvula) And at least one of the following: a. Respiratory compromise (e.g., dyspnea, wheeze-bronchospasm, stridor, reduced PEF, hypoxemia); b. Reduced BP or associated symptoms of end-organ dysfunction (e.g., hypotonia [collapse], syncope, incontinence); c. Severe gastrointestinal symptoms (e.g., severe crampy abdominal pain, repetitive vomiting), especially after exposure to non-food allergens.

Criteria	Characterization of symptoms [NIAID/FAAN, 2005]	Characterization of symptoms [WAOAG, 2020]
2	Two or more of the following occur rapidly after exposure to a likely allergen for that patient (minutes to several hours): a. Involvement of the skin-mucosal tissue (e.g., generalized hives, itch-flush, swollen lips-tongue-uvula); b. Respiratory compromise (e.g., dyspnea, wheeze-bronchospasm, stridor, reduced PEF, hypoxemia); c. Reduced BP or associated symptoms (e.g., hypotonia [collapse], syncope, incontinence); d. Persistent gastrointestinal symptoms (e.g., crampy abdominal pain, vomiting).	Acute onset of hypotension* or bronchospasm** or laryngeal involvement*** after exposure to a known or highly probable allergen**** for that patient (minutes to several hours), even in the absence of typical skin involvement.
3	Reduced BP after exposure to known allergen for that patient (minutes to several hours): a. Infants and children: low systolic BP (age specific) or greater than 30% decrease in systolic BP*; b. Adults: systolic BP of less than 90 mm Hg or greater than 30% decrease from that person's baseline.	
	PEF, Peak expiratory flow; BP, blood pressure. **Low systolic blood pressure for children is defined as less than 70 mm Hg from 1 month to 1 year, less than (70 mm Hg1[23age]) from 1 to 10 years, and less than 90 mm Hg from 11 to 17 years.*	*PEF, Peak expiratory flow; BP, blood pressure.* **Hypotension is defined as a decrease in systolic BP greater than 30% from that person's baseline, or* *i. Infants and children under 10 years: systolic BP less than (70 mm Hgþ [2 x age in years])* *ii. Adults and children over 10 years: systolic BP less than<90 mmHg.* *** Excluding lower respiratory symptoms triggered by common inhalant allergens or food allergens perceived to cause "inhalational" reactions in the absence of ingestion.* ****Laryngeal symptoms include stridor, vocal changes, and odynophagia.* *****An allergen is a substance (usually a protein) capable of triggering an immune response that can result in an allergic reaction. Most allergens act through an IgE-mediated pathway, but some non-allergen triggers can act independent of IgE (e.g., via direct activation of mast cells).*

Table 2.
Clinical criteria for diagnosis of anaphylaxis (anaphylaxis is highly likely when any one of the following criteria is fulfilled).

Anaphylaxis Network (NIAID/FAAN) [47] and the new 2020 clinical criteria of World Allergy Organization Anaphylaxis Guidance (WAOAG) [1] are used (**Table 2**). The distinctive feature of WAOAG criteria is the possibility of diagnosing anaphylaxis if an isolated potentially life-threatening bronchospasm or laryngeal involvement symptoms develop in response to allergen exposure. Such an approach helps to increase the verification rate of anaphylaxis diagnosis since isolated cases of acute life-threatening allergic reactions deserve special attention according to most studies [48, 49]. According to our practice, the 2020 criteria are particularly relevant in pediatric or intensive care units providing emergency medical treatment.

Evaluation of anaphylaxis symptoms in infants in terms of existing criteria is often challenging, as it requires knowledge of the relevant nosology and clinical experience. In addition to the acknowledged symptoms of anaphylaxis, such as skin manifestations, problems with respiratory and cardiovascular system, gastrointestinal disorders, and behavioral reactions typical for infants are described by parents in many ways: "falling asleep," "goes limp," etc. Symptom descriptions can sometimes be influenced by national colloquialisms that are difficult for the physician to understand. For example, in Russia, parents sometimes describe their child's falling asleep with the term "to nod off," which is not at all associated with this symptom in other languages. Some children with anaphylaxis have rarer symptoms, such as hoarseness of voice, dysphonia, salivation, constant crying, and weeping. Studies covering the diagnosis of anaphylaxis in infants are sparse, but even based on the few data, some age-dependent features of the clinical pattern of anaphylaxis can be traced. It is highly likely that there is a connection between the trigger, shock organ involvement, and the severity of the reaction.

4.2 Clinical presentation and differential diagnosis of anaphylaxis in infants

Skin and mucous tissue manifestations are the most common for anaphylaxis in infants. According to most studies, the incidence of these anaphylaxis symptoms can be as high as 98–100% [11, 13]. This group of symptoms includes urticaria (usually generalized), erythema (more often multiforme), angioedema, and contact urticaria (infrequent, e.g., after contact with allergen). Retrospectively, photographs and questions to parents about skin manifestations are helpful: how quickly the rash appeared after exposure; how long the rash lasted; whether the rash was similar to the previous episodes; whether there was itching and other sensations; and where the rash was located. It is necessary to find out whether the child had a fever at the time the symptoms appeared, whether there were any other symptoms typical for infectious diseases, at what time of the day the rash appeared, etc. These questions will help to objectify clinical symptoms and rule out diseases not associated with systemic reactions (e.g., viral exanthem, mastocytosis, various forms of contact dermatitis).

Respiratory tract symptoms, along with skin manifestations of anaphylaxis in infants, more often rank second in incidence. However, in several studies, the incidence of respiratory symptoms of anaphylaxis in infants varies considerably and ranges from 48 to 98% [7, 8, 11, 17, 20, 21, 50]. Respiratory signs of anaphylactic reactions in infants include cough, stridor, wheeze, difficulties with inhalation and/or exhalation, rhinorrhea, and oropharyngeal symptoms (dysphonia, hoarseness/loss of voice, problems with swallowing). Several comparative studies demonstrated a significantly lower incidence of wheeze, cough, and dyspnea symptoms of anaphylaxis in infants compared with the older age group [7, 20, 22]. According to our data collected Russia, cough was observed in 73% of cases of food-induced anaphylaxis in infants [13]. However, cough associated with food intake can be due to many causes (e.g., introduction of complementary food of denser consistency, regurgitation, aspiration), which should be considered when evaluating this symptom in the diagnosis of anaphylaxis.

Gastrointestinal tract symptoms are particularly typical for the clinical picture of anaphylaxis in infants. As observed by Topal et al. [11], in children in the first year of life, the frequency of gastrointestinal symptoms in the form of persistent vomiting reaches 30.4%, which, for example, is half as frequent (14.8%) in children over 1-year-old. Pouessel et al. [20] note that the rate of gastrointestinal anaphylaxis symptoms in infants <1 year of age is 49%, yielding only to skin and mucous membrane manifestations. According to the results of our investigation conducted in Russia among infants <1 year of age, in case of anaphylactic reactions after consumption of cow's milk, the frequency of gastrointestinal system involvement amounted to 53% and was many times higher, in comparison with the group of patients older than 1-year-old (11%) [51]. Such data emphasize the relevance of gastrointestinal symptoms as an important clinical criterion for the diagnosis of anaphylaxis in infants. However, the differential search should consider that vomiting and abdominal pain are quite common in infants and may be associated with refluxes, constipation, infections, acute surgical diseases, non-IgE-mediated allergic diseases, etc.

Cardiovascular symptoms in anaphylaxis are less common in infants. According to our observation and most studies, their incidence varies from 7 to 21% [8, 11, 20, 51]. One reason for the variability in the incidence of these symptoms is the frequent absence of blood pressure monitoring, and perhaps this examination is the most infrequent in such patients [52]. According to a study conducted at the pediatric emergency department in New York, only 12.5% of patients under 3 years of age had their blood pressure measured, compared with 90% of children above 3 years old [12, 53]. According to the study of Turkish colleagues, blood pressure in anaphylactic reactions was measured in only 21.7% of first-year infants, compared with 54.3% of patients older than 1 year of age [11]. The observed low incidence of cardiovascular anaphylaxis in this group of patients is often related to the lack of appropriate equipment, the necessary size of the tonometer cuff, and the difficulties with measuring blood pressure if the child is anxious. It should be emphasized that it is important not only to measure blood pressure once but also to monitor this indicator. In infants, hypotension is a late clinical sign indicating decreased tissue perfusion and decompensated shock, so it is crucial to diagnose anaphylaxis and start treatment, to recognize the earliest cardiovascular symptoms of shock: pallor, marbling, skin cyanosis, lethargy, hypotension, tachypnoea, increasing tachycardia (in the absence of crying) [54].

Thus, there are a number of circumstances that significantly complicate the diagnosis of anaphylaxis in the group of young children: the first episode of anaphylaxis, the presence of not clearly expressed and quickly disappearing symptoms, infants cannot describe symptoms and actively present complaints, so a number of subjective manifestations (itching, pain, sensations, etc.) cannot be assessed, the presence of nonspecific symptoms (crying, screaming, etc.) is extremely difficult to interpret, there are technical difficulties of objectification and monitoring. In this situation, the doctor's attention should be focused on finding out the contact with the suspected allergen, usually food in the case of infants.

Standardized criteria are used to assess the severity of anaphylactic reactions [55]. It is determined by the most affected organ system, but it is extremely difficult in the case of infants. Information about fatal anaphylaxis in the pediatric population is extremely limited and variable, and in general incidence does not exceed 1% [56]. Von Starck et al. [57] for the first time describe the fatal outcome of food-induced anaphylaxis of a boy aged 1.5 years. The child suffered from atopic eczema and had three episodes of generalized allergic reactions after eating several spoonfuls of mashed peas. After that, a provocation test with this product was carried out in the hospital, during which angioedema, cyanosis, and collapse developed. The boy died despite resuscitation. There are no reliable data on specific risk factors predisposing to fatal/almost fatal anaphylaxis in infants.

4.3 Laboratory diagnosis

Currently, there are no universal laboratory markers that can diagnose anaphylaxis with high probability, but some markers may be useful to confirm the diagnosis and determine the trigger. Practically applicable nonspecific tests include the determination of tryptase concentration in blood in the time interval from 15 minutes to 3 hours after the first symptoms of anaphylaxis and the dynamics after the anaphylaxis episode (basal tryptase level). It should be considered that the normal level of total tryptase among children <6–9 months of age is higher than among older children, adolescents, and adults. Thus, the average level of tryptase among children <3 months of age with hereditary predisposition to allergy is 14.2 ± 10.2 mg/l, while among healthy children it is 6.13 ± 3.47 mg/l [58]. With age, there is a gradual decrease in the level of tryptase, and only by 9–12 months of life, it reaches normal reference values (3.85 ± 1.8 mg/l), which can be objectively interpreted. Data from one study demonstrated elevated levels of β-tryptase in the blood of deceased patients diagnosed with sudden infant death syndrome (SIDS) [59]. Therefore, the authors suggest the possibility of undiagnosed anaphylaxis cases in infants disguised as SIDS. The results of another similar study were mixed [60]. Importantly, in the presence of an appropriate clinical pattern, low or normal tryptase levels do not exclude the diagnosis of anaphylaxis; this marker is most informative for drug, perioperative, and insect anaphylaxis and to a lesser extent for its other types.

To detect sensitization and to trigger anaphylaxis, the determination of specific IgE immunoglobulin using the ImmunoCap test system and the immuno solid-phase allergy chip (ISAC) is optimal in most cases, and these methods are highly informative. When performing allergy testing in infants, it should be borne in mind that even minimal detectable sensitization can be significant for the development of anaphylaxis. According to our observation, almost all patients with food-induced anaphylaxis, including infants, were able to detect sensitization to allergen; its level varied greatly (from threshold (≥0.35 kU/L) to maximum (>100 KU/L) (ImmunoCap, Phadia, Sweden) and did not correlate with the severity of reactions [13]. A certain degree of correlation was found only between specific IgE levels >100 KU/L to fish/seafood allergens and inhalation hypersensitivity inducing anaphylaxis by inhaling the allergen (e.g., cooking and cutting fish) [38, 61]. Jeon et al. [7] demonstrate that more than 90% of children with anaphylaxis to hen's egg <24 months of age and all children >2 years of age had sensitization to this allergen above DDP (95% decision points). However, specific IgE levels in cow's milk exceeded DDP only in less than half of the children with anaphylaxis to this allergen. Therefore, in case of negative allergy tests, but with a convincing history of anaphylaxis, it is necessary to repeat allergy testing over time. According to the research, the ISAC platform can be particularly useful in identifying triggers in patients with idiopathic anaphylaxis [62].

5. Treatment

Treatment of anaphylaxis in infants is completely based on the recommendations and principles of therapy of anaphylactic reactions in older patients (**Figure 1**) [58].

In case of anaphylaxis, treatment should begin immediately with a written protocol. It is necessary to stop receiving any suspected trigger (e.g., food and medication); evaluate blood circulation, skin, airway, breathing, age, and body weight; call the emergency medical service for help. Place the infant supine or semi reclining in a

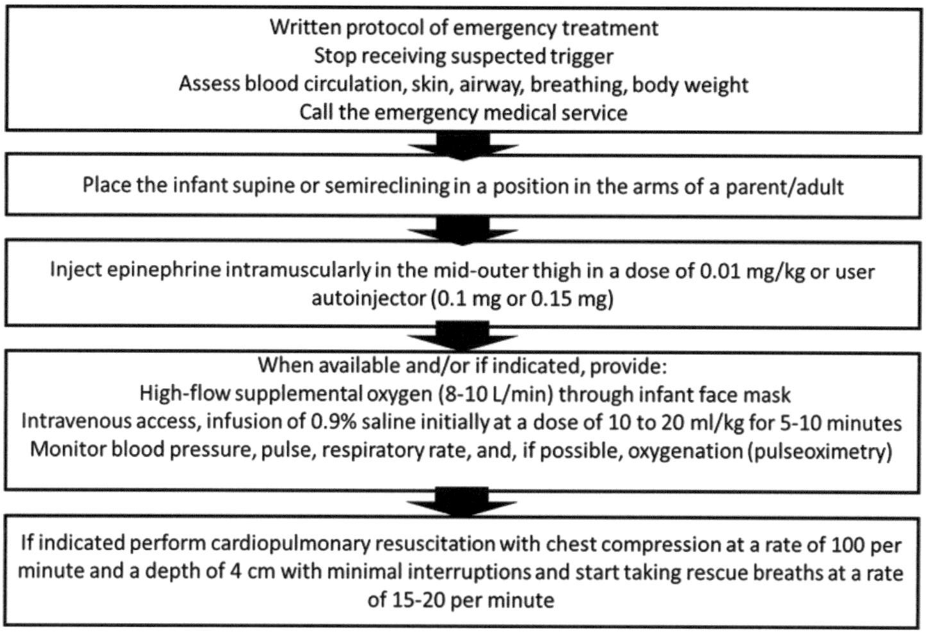

Figure 1.
Algorithm for the treatment of anaphylaxis in infants, data from Simons et al. [58].

position in the arms of a parent/adult (not upright over the shoulder) and immediately inject epinephrine intramuscularly in the mid-outer thigh. Anaphylaxis is an absolute indication for the administration of epinephrine (the first-choice drug), the recommended initial dose is 0.01 mg/kg intramuscularly. If there is no effect from the first dose, second administration is possible after 5–10 min. It is important that infants with anaphylaxis can remain pale despite 2–3 doses of epinephrine, so persistent pallor in itself is not a sign of poor treatment effectiveness and an indication for an increase in the dose of epinephrine, it should be interpreted taking into account blood pressure and other symptoms monitoring. In addition, more than 2–3 doses of epinephrine in infants can cause hypertension and tachycardia, tachycardia may be mistakenly interpreted as a continuing cardiovascular symptom of anaphylaxis [63]. When injecting epinephrine (especially when using an autoinjector) into an infant, it is necessary to fix the limb, this avoids traumatization and ensures the correct administration of epinephrine. After the injection of epinephrine, it is impossible to verticalize the patient's position (e.g., to sit down or get up), because this can lead to a fatal outcome within a few seconds. Most countries have registered autoinjectors for children weighing more than 15 kg in two fixed doses of epinephrine: 0.15 mg and 0.3 mg. Most infants weigh less than 10–15 kg; however, autoinjector containing the third dose of epinephrine - 0.1 mg was approved in November 2017 by Food and Drug Administration in the USA, but so far it is not available everywhere, which makes it difficult to administer the dose prescribed in the protocol for this category of patients. Using an epinephrine autoinjector with a dose of 0.15 mg for infants weighing 7.5 kg provides up to 200% of the recommended dose at a rate of 0.01 mg/kg [64, 65]. However, administering epinephrine *via* autoinjector presents less risk than using epinephrine syringes and ampoules, where dosing errors and delays in administration increase the potential risk, especially in the absence of medical training. Another widely debated issue is the needle length of existing autoinjectors because it is not always suitable for intramuscular injection in infants. According to Kim et al. [66] who performed an ultrasound assessment of the distance from the surface to the thigh bone in 53 children (mean age 18.9 months, mean body weight 11 kg), it was found that using the existing autoinjector length of 12.7 mm (autoinjector 0.15 mg) in 43.1% of patients could lead to intraosseous infusion. Thus, there are quite significant difficulties for physicians when prescribing epinephrine to infants, which significantly reduces the frequency of its use. According to Fleischer et al. [67], only 29.9% of patients in the first 2 years of life use epinephrine to relieve symptoms of severe anaphylaxis. The researchers note that the reasons caregivers do not prescribe epinephrine are difficulty in recognizing the severity of anaphylaxis, lack of epinephrine, and problems associated with administering it. Similar findings were reported by colleagues in France, where only ¼ of patients under 1 year of age with food-induced anaphylaxis had injections of epinephrine, in none of these cases autoinjectors were used [20]. Research in Korea and Turkey demonstrated a higher rate of epinephrine administration in children under 12 months of age (46.8% and 40.6%, respectively) [7, 22]. According to our observation conducted in Russia, the frequency of prescribing epinephrine in infants to relieve symptoms of anaphylaxis 10 years ago did not exceed 7%; currently, there is a positive trend of higher incidence of prescribing epinephrine (21%) [13, 68].

Depending on the severity of the detected symptoms and the level of medical capabilities according to the indications additionally provided: high-flow oxygen supply through a facial infant mask (8–10 L /min); intravenous access and infusion of 0.9% saline initially at a dose of 10 to 20 ml/kg for 5–10 minutes. It is mandatory to monitor blood pressure, pulse, respiratory rate, and, if possible, oxygenation by using pulse oximetry. In the absence of a monitor to measure blood pressure, the pulse is counted manually every 2–5 minutes. You should be ready to perform cardiopulmonary resuscitation with chest compression at a rate of 100 per minute and a depth of 4 cm with minimal interruptions and start taking rescue breaths at a rate of 15–20 per minute [58].

The use of other adjuvant medications (H1-antihistamines, glucocorticosteroids, colloidal solutions, etc.) and additional therapeutic and diagnostic manipulations (oxygen support, measurement of blood pressure, resuscitation, etc.) to control the symptoms of anaphylaxis in infants is performed as per indications while respecting the advised doses of drugs, the algorithm of first aid in case of anaphylaxis in elderly patients. Although no adjuvant medication replaces epinephrine, antihistamines and glucocorticosteroids continue to be the predominant drugs by frequency of use in controlling the symptoms of anaphylaxis. Importantly, first-generation H1-antihistamines in common doses can cause sedation and conceal several symptoms, which may impede the diagnosis of anaphylaxis. In addition, their parenteral use can lead to a respiratory arrest in young children, as well as lower blood pressure, which justifies their use in anaphylaxis only when blood pressure is normal [69, 70].

In cases of anaphylaxis or suspected anaphylaxis in infants, admission to the intensive care unit and symptom monitoring for at least 24 hours is necessary. This recommendation is critically important for patients with severe or prolonged anaphylaxis (e.g., repeated doses of epinephrine or intravenous infusions are required), including in the anamnesis; if the patient has concomitant diseases (e.g., severe asthma, arrhythmia, mastocytosis); if the patient lives away from medical care; if anaphylaxis has developed in the evening or at night.

After a case of anaphylaxis, the patient should be prescribed epinephrine (autoinjector or syringe and ampoule) and clear recommendations should be given for its administration. Moreover, currently, there are absolute and relative indications for prescribing self-injectable epinephrine in childhood, including children, who have not yet experienced anaphylaxis, but have a high risk of anaphylaxis, [71, 72]. **Table 3**. In our experience, among the absolutely presented indications for prescribing self-injectable epinephrine in infants, the most relevant are as follows: any history of anaphylaxis (including idiopathic anaphylaxis); food allergy and coexisting persistent asthma; previous cardiovascular or respiratory reaction to a food, especially in combination with gastrointestinal and skin/mucosal tissue symptoms. Among the relative presented indications for prescribing self-injectable epinephrine in infants, the most relevant are as follows: any reaction to small amounts of food (e.g., airborne food allergen or contact only *via* skin); history of only a previous mild reaction to peanut or a tree nut; high sensitization to specific food triggers known to be associated with severe/fatal reactions (e.g., peanut, tree nut, seafood, and milk); remoteness of home from medical facilities; certain comorbidities (asthma, mastocytosis). There are no absolute contraindications to administering epinephrine in children, because children usually do not suffer from any serious concomitant diseases, such as coronary heart disease or cardiac arrhythmias. If an infant with anaphylaxis has a high risk of tachyarrhythmias, the doctor should weigh the risks and benefits and take into account that epinephrine in anaphylaxis can save lives. Data from a number of studies [73–75] demonstrate that

Absolute indications [71]	**Relative indications [71]**
• Previous cardiovascular or respiratory reaction to a food, insect sting, or latex • Exercise-induced anaphylaxis • Idiopathic anaphylaxis • Child with food allergy and coexistent persistent asthma* **This is an opinion-based indication extrapolated from data emerging from retrospective studies.*	• Any reaction to small amounts of food (e.g., airborne food allergen or contact only via skin) • History of only a previous mild reaction to peanut or a tree nut • Remoteness of home from medical facilities • Food allergic reaction in a teenager

Examples of factors that may indicate the need to prescribe epinephrine for persons "at risk" of anaphylaxis [72]*
Reaction history • Reaction to trace allergen exposure. • Repeat exposures likely. • Specific food triggers are known to be associated with severe/fatal reactions (e.g., peanut, tree nut, seafood, and milk). • Generalized urticaria from insect venom. **Certain comorbidities:** • Asthma • Use of nonselective β-blockers. **Additional factors:** • Initial reaction details unclear, possible anaphylaxis. • Those living in a remote area away from medical care/access. **An at-risk person can be, for example, one with a confirmed allergy to food or insect venom who has not experienced anaphylaxis. Note: the first episode of anaphylaxis can be fatal.*

Table 3.
Indications for prescribing self-injectable epinephrine, data from Muraro A et al. [71], Sicherer S et al. [72].

up to 20% of patients with anaphylaxis need a second dose of epinephrine; in addition, one dose may not be enough to prevent the fatal outcome of anaphylaxis in some patients. In this regard, as a rule, the patient (the patient's parents) is recommended to have two epinephrine autoinjectors, this is due to a number of factors: the possibility of a misfire, remote residence from emergency medical care, a large body weight of the child (e.g., >45 kg), lack of effect from the first dose of epinephrine in the anamnesis, biphasic anaphylaxis, etc.

Allergy examination should be performed on all children with suspected anaphylaxis at allergy clinics with experience in the management of such patients. Information about anaphylaxis, and its causal factors (food, medication, insect sting, etc.) should always be available and accompany the patient, for example, indicated on a special medallion, bracelet, or clothing (e.g., t-shirts). Adults (parents, caregivers, teachers, etc.) surrounding the child with a history of anaphylactic reactions should be thoroughly informed about the diagnosis of anaphylaxis, the features of the clinical picture of its development, and a plan of emergency action, including mandatory administration of epinephrine. Particular attention should be paid to the exclusion of repeated episodes of anaphylaxis. In the group of infants <1 year of age, these reactions can be associated not only with misleading food labels and accidental contamination with allergen but also with deliberate attempts to expand the child's diet and introduction of previously excluded products to which children have been sensitized. Nowadays, there are training sessions on anaphylaxis (schools, online training, etc.) that help to significantly reduce anxiety in the family, because the presence of a child with this diagnosis provokes a state of fear for his life, due to the inability to provide timely treatment.

6. Conclusions

Thus, for young children, there are features of the triggers' spectrum and clinical manifestations of anaphylaxis, which should be considered when making a diagnosis, and to improve the existing clinical criteria of anaphylaxis in future. The development and availability of new types of autoinjectors for safe administration of epinephrine to small patients and the development of new therapeutic strategies for anaphylaxis are essential. The search for potential specific markers/predictors of anaphylaxis, applicable in routine practice to allow timely diagnosis of anaphylaxis and formation of a risk group before the development of a life-threatening situation, which is especially important for children in the first years of life, is relevant.

Conflict of interest

The authors declare no conflict of interest.

Author details

Natalia Esakova[1*], Alexander Nikolaevich Pampura[1], Nazifa Dustbabaeva[2] and Venera Baybekova[2]

1 Veltischev Research and Clinical Institute for Pediatrics and Pediatric Surgery of the Pirogov Russian National Research Medical University of the Russian Ministry of Health, Moscow, Russia

2 Republican Scientific and Specialized Allergological Center of the Ministry of Health of the Republic of Uzbekistan, Tashkent, Uzbekistan

*Address all correspondence to: envoo7@rambler.ru

References

[1] Cardona V, Ansotegui IJ, Ebisawa M, El-Gamal Y, Rivas MF, Fineman S, et al. World allergy organization anaphylaxis guidance, 2020. World Allergy Organization Journal. 2020;**13**(10): 100472

[2] Young MC. General treatment of anaphylaxis. In: Leung DYM, Sampson HA, Geha RS, Szefler SJ, editors. Pediatric Allergy Principles and Practice. St Louis (MO): Mosby, Inc; 2003. pp. 643-654

[3] Simons FE, Chad ZH, Gold M. Anaphylaxis in children: Real-time reporting from a national network. Allergy Clinical Immunology. 2004;**1**:242

[4] Mehl A, Wahn U, Niggemann B. Anaphylactic reactions in children: A questionnaire-based survey in Germany. Allergy. 2005;**60**:1440-1445

[5] Tejedor Alonso MA, Moro MM, Hernandez JE, Mugica Garcia MV, Albelda CV, Ingelmo AR, et al. Incidence of anaphylaxis in hospitalized patients. International Archives of Allergy and Immunology. 2011;**156**:212-220

[6] Poulos LM, Waters AM, Correll PK, Loblay RH, Marks GB. Trends in hospitalizations for anaphylaxis, angioedema, and urticaria in Australia, 1993-1994 to 2004-2005. The Journal of Allergy and Clinical Immunology. 2007;**120**:878-884

[7] Jeon YH, Lee S, Ahn K, Lee SY, Kim KY, Kim HH, et al. Infantile anaphylaxis in Korea: A multicenter retrospective case study. Journal of Korean Medical Science. 2019;**34**(13):e106

[8] Rudders SA, Banerji A, Clark S, Camargo CA Jr. Age-related differences in the clinical presentation of food-induced anaphylaxis. The Journal of Pediatrics. 2011;**158**(2):326-328

[9] Samady W, Trainor J, Smith B, Gupta R. Food-induced anaphylaxis in infants and children. Annals of Allergy, Asthma & Immunology. 2018;**121**(3):360-365

[10] Silva R, Gomes E, Cunha L, Falcão H. Anaphylaxis in children: A nine years retrospective study (2001-2009). Allergology Immunopathology (Madr). 2012;**40**(1):31-36

[11] Topal E, Bakirtas A, Yilmaz O, Ertoy Karagol IH, Arga M, Demirsoy MS, et al. Anaphylaxis in infancy compared with older children. Allergy and Asthma Proceedings. 2013;**34**:233-238

[12] Huang F, Chawla K, Jarvinen KM, Nowak-Węgrzyn A. Anaphylaxis in a New York City pediatric emergency department: Triggers, treatments, and outcomes. The Journal of Allergy and Clinical Immunology. 2012;**129**(1):162-168

[13] Esakova NV, Treneva MS, Okuneva TS, Pampura AN. Food anaphylaxis: Reported cases in Russian Federation Children. American Journal of Public Health Research. 2015;**5**:187-191

[14] Motosue MS, Bellolio MF, Van Houten HK, Shah ND, Campbell RL. Increasing emergency department visits for anaphylaxis, 2005-2014. The Journal of Allergy and Clinical Immunology. In Practice. 2017;**5**:171-175

[15] Dyer AA, Lau CH, Smith TL, Smith BM, Gupta RS. Pediatric emergency department visits and hospitalizations due to food-induced

anaphylaxis in Illinois. Annals of Allergy, Asthma & Immunology. 2015;**115**(1):56-62

[16] Pampura AN, Esakova NV. Anafilaksiya u detej. M.: ID MEDPRAKTIKA. 2020. p. 368

[17] Jiang X. Xiang Age-related differences in characteristics of anaphylaxis in Chinese children from infancy to adolescence. World Allergy Organization Journal. 2021;**14**:100605

[18] Speakman S, Kool B, Sinclair J, Fitzharris P. Paediatric food-induced anaphylaxis hospital presentations in New Zealand. Journal of Paediatrics and Child Health. 2018;**54**:254-259

[19] Goh SH, Soh JY, Loh W, Lee KP, Tan SC, Heng WJK, et al. Cause and Clinical Presentation of Anaphylaxis in Singapore: From Infancy to Old Age. International Archives of Allergy and Immunology. 2018;**175**:91-98

[20] Pouessel G, Jean-Bart C, Deschildre A, Van der Brempt X, Tanno LK, Beaumont P, et al. Food-induced anaphylaxis in infancy compared to preschool age: A retrospective analysis. Clinical and Experimental Allergy. 2020;**50**(1):74-81

[21] Ko J, Zhu S, Alabaster A, Wang J, Sax DR. Prehospital treatment and emergency department outcomes in young children with food allergy. The Journal of Allergy and Clinical Immunology. 2020;**8**:2302-2309

[22] Kahveci M, Akarsu A, Koken G, Sahiner UM, Soyer O, Sekerel BE. Food-induced anaphylaxis in infants, as compared to toddlers and preschool children in Turkey. Pediatric Allergy and Immunology. 2020;**31**(8):954-961

[23] Andrew E, Nehme Z, Bernard S, Smith K. Pediatric anaphylaxis in the prehospital setting: Incidence, characteristics, and management. Prehospital Emergency Care. 2018;**22**(4):445-451

[24] Alvarez-Perea A, Ameiro B, Morales C, Zambrano G, Rodríguez A, Guzmán M, et al. Anaphylaxis in the pediatric emergency department: Analysis of 133 cases after an allergy workup. The Journal of Allergy and Clinical Immunology. In Practice. 2017;**5**(5):1256-1263

[25] Rajani PS, Martin H, Groetch M, Järvinen KM. Presentation and management of food allergy in breastfed infants and risks of maternal elimination diets. The Journal of Allergy and Clinical Immunology. In Practice. 2020;**8**(1):52-67

[26] Monti G, Marinaro L, Libanore V, Peltran A, Muratore MC, Silvestro L. Anaphylaxis due to fish hypersensitivity in an exclusively breastfed infant. Acta Paediatrica. 2006;**95**(11):1514-1515

[27] Arima T, Campos-Alberto E, Funakoshi H, Inoue Y, Tomiita M, Kohno Y, et al. Immediate systemic allergic reaction in an infant to fish allergen ingested through breast milk. Asia Pacific Allergy. 2016;**6**(4):257-259

[28] Lifschitz CH, Hawkins HK, Guerra C, Byrd N. Anaphylactic shock due to cow's milk protein hypersensitivity in a breast-fed infant. Journal of Pediatric Gastroenterology and Nutrition. 1988;**7**(1):141-144

[29] Ammar F, de Boissieu D, Dupont C. Allergy to protein hydrolysates. Report of 30 cases. Archives de Pédiatrie. 1999;**6**(8):837-843

[30] Horino S, Satou T, Nihei M, Miura K. Slow oral immunotherapy for cow's milk allergy with anaphylaxis to extensively

hydrolyzed formula. Pediatrics and Neonatology. 2020;**61**(3):355-356

[31] Cantani A, Micera M. Allergenicity of a whey hypoallergenic formula in genetically at risk babies: Four case reports. European Review for Medical and Pharmacological Sciences. 2005;**9**:179-182

[32] Pessler F, Nejat M. Anaphylactic reaction to goat's milk in a cow's milk-allergic infant. Pediatric Allergy and Immunology. 2004;**15**:183-185

[33] De Swert LF, Cadot P, Ceuppens JL. Diagnosis and natural course of allergy to cooked potatoes in children. Allergy. 2007;**62**:750-757

[34] Dalal I, Binson I, Levine A, Somekh E, Ballin A, Reifen R. The pattern of sesame sensitivity among infants and children. Pediatric Allergy and Immunology. 2003;**14**:312-316

[35] Roberts JR, Gerstner TV, Grewar DA. Allergy to caribou and seal meats in Inuit children: A report of three cases. The Journal of Allergy and Clinical Immunology. 2006;**117**:S42

[36] Tuncel T, Uysal P, Hocaoglu AB, Erge DO, Firinci F, Karaman O, et al. Anaphylaxis caused by honey ingestion in an infant. Allergologia et Immunopathologia. 2011;**39**:112-113

[37] Zurzolo GA, Allen KJ, Peters RL, Tang ML, Dharmage S, de Courten M, et al. Anaphylaxis to packaged foods in Australasia. Journal of Paediatrics and Child Health. 2018;**54**(5):551-555

[38] Esakova NV, Pampura AN. Features of food anaphylaxis in children arising from alternative routes of allergen intake. Pediatria n.a. G.N. Speransky. 2021;**100**(2):57-63

[39] Xing Y, Zhang H, Sun S, Ma X, Pleasants Roy A, Tan H, et al. Clinical features and treatment of pediatric patients with drug-induced anaphylaxis: A study based on pharmacovigilance data. European Journal of Pediatrics. 2018;**177**:145-154

[40] Gabrielli S, Clarke AE, Eisman H, Morris J, Joseph L, La Vieille S, et al. Disparities in rate, triggers, and management in pediatric and adult cases of suspected drug-induced anaphylaxis in Canada. Immunity, Inflammation and Disease. 2018;**6**:3-12

[41] Moneret-Vautrin DA, Morisset M, Cordebar V, Codréanu F, Kanny G. Probiotics may be unsafe in infants allergic to cow's milk. Allergy. 2006;**61**:507-508

[42] McNeil MM, Weintraub ES, Duffy J, Sukumaran L, Jacobsen SJ, Klein NP. Risk of anaphylaxis after vaccination in children and adults. The Journal of Allergy and Clinical Immunology. 2016;**137**:868-878

[43] Yavuz ST, Sahiner UM, Sekerel BE, Tuncer A, Kalayci O, Sackesen C. Anaphylactic reactions to measles-mumps-rubella vaccine in three children with allergies to hen's egg and cow's milk. Acta Paediatrica. 2011;**100**:94-96

[44] Dreskin SC, Halsey NA, Kelso JM, Wood RA, Hummell DS, Edwards KM, et al. International Consensus (ICON): Allergic reactions to vaccines. World Allergy Organ Journal. 2016;**9**:32

[45] Kelso JM, Jones RT, Yunginger JW. Anaphylaxis to measles, mumps, and rubella vaccine mediated by IgE to gelatin. The Journal of Allergy and Clinical Immunology. 1993;**91**:867-872

[46] Lee JM, Greenes DS. Biphasic anaphylactic reactions in pediatrics. Pediatrics. 2000;**106**:762-766

[47] Sampson HA, Munoz-Furlong A, Campbell RL, et al. Second symposium on the definition and management of anaphylaxis: Summary report – Second national institute of allergy and infectious disease/food allergy and anaphylaxis network symposium. Journal of Allergy Clinical Immunology. 2005;**117**:391-397

[48] Greenberger PA, Rotskoff BD, Lifschultz B. Fatal anaphylaxis: Postmortem findings and associated comorbid diseases. Annals of Allergy, Asthma & Immunology. 2007;**98**(3):252-257

[49] Pumphrey R, Sturm G. Risk factors for fatal anaphylaxis. In: Moneret-Vautrin DA, editor. Advances in Anaphylaxis Management. London: Future Medicine; 2014. pp. 32-48

[50] Lee S. Food allergy and food-induced anaphylaxis in children: An increasing critical public health issue. Korean Journal of Pediatrics. 2019;**62**(12):431-432

[51] Esakova NV, Pampura AN, Varlamov EE. Anafilaksiya k moloku u detej. Voprosy detskoj dietologii. 2014;**12**(1):39-42

[52] Simons FE, Ardusso LR, et al. International consensus on (ICON) anaphylaxis. World Allergy Organ Journal. 2014;**30**:7-9

[53] Dosanjh A. Infant anaphylaxis: The importance of early recognition. Journal of Asthma Allergy. 2013;**6**:103-107

[54] Pistiner M, Handorff A, Camargo CA Jr, Cohen A. Cardiovascular symptoms/signs in infants and toddlers with anaphylaxis. The Journal of Allergy and Clinical Immunology. In Practice. 2021;**9**:1044-1046

[55] Sampson HA. Anaphylaxis and emergency treatment. Pediatrics. 2003;**111**:1601-1608

[56] Ramsey NB, Guffey D, Anagnostou K, Coleman NE, Davis CM. Epidemiology of anaphylaxis in critically ill children in the United States and Canada. Journal of Allergy Clinical Immunology Practise. 2019;**7**:2241-2219

[57] Von Starck K. Primäre spezifische Allergie und idiosynkratischer Schock. Monatsschrift für Kinderheilkunde. 1926;**32**:119-127

[58] Simons FE, Sampson HA. Anaphylaxis: Unique aspects of clinical diagnosis and management in infants (birth to age 2 years). The Journal of Allergy and Clinical Immunology. 2015;**5**:1125-1131

[59] Buckley MG, Variend S, Walls AF. Elevated serum concentrations of beta-tryptase, but not alpha-tryptase, in Sudden Infant Death Syndrome (SIDS). An investigation of anaphylactic mechanisms. Clinical Experience in Allergy. 2001;**31**:1696-1704

[60] Hagan LL, Goetz DW, Revercomb CH, Garriott J. Sudden infant death syndrome: A search for allergen hypersensitivity. Annals of Allergy, Asthma & Immunology. 1998;**80**:227-231

[61] Esakova NV, Pampura AN, Varlamov EE, Okuneva TS. Clinical and immunological features of anaphylaxis to fish in children. Experimental and Clinical Gastroenterology. 2017;**1**:78-82

[62] Heaps A, Carter S, Selwood C, Moody M, Unsworth J, Deacock S, et al. The utility of the ISAC allergen array in the investigation of idiopathic anaphylaxis. Clinical and Experimental Immunology. 2014;**177**:483-490

[63] Simons FE. Anaphylaxis in infants: Can recognition and management be improved? The Journal of Allergy and Clinical Immunology. 2007;**120**:537-540

[64] Brown JC. Epinephrine, auto-injectors, and anaphylaxis: Challenges of dose, depth, and device. Annals of Allergy, Asthma & Immunology. 2018;**121**:53-60

[65] Frith K, Smith J, Joshi P, Ford LS, Vale S. Updated anaphylaxis guidelines: Management in infants and children. Australian Prescriber. 2021;**44**:91-95

[66] Kim H, Dinakar C, McInnis P, Rudin D, Benain X, Daley W, et al. Inadequacy of current pediatric epinephrine autoinjector needle length for use in infants and toddlers. Annals of Allergy, Asthma & Immunology. 2017;**118**:719-725

[67] Fleischer DM, Perry TT, Atkins D, Wood RA, Burks AW, Jones SM, et al. Allergic reactions to foods in preschoolaged children in a prospective observational food allergy study. Pediatrics. 2012;**130**:e25-e32. DOI: 10.1542/peds.2011-1762

[68] Esakova NV, Zakharova IN, Osmanov IM, Kolushkin DS, Pampura AN. Anaphylaxis among children hospitalized with severe allergic reactions: A 5-year retrospective analysis. Pediatrics. 2022;**20**:21-30

[69] Sheikh A, Broek VM, Brown SGA, Simons FER. H1-antihistamines for the treatment of anaphylaxis with and without shock. Cochrane Database of Systematic Reviews. 2007;**1**:CD006160

[70] Starke PR, Weaver J, Chowdhury BA. Boxed warning added to promethazine labeling for pediatric use. The New England Journal of Medicine. 2005;**352**:2653

[71] Muraro A, Roberts G, Clark A, Eigenmann PA, Halken S, Lack G, et al. The management of anaphylaxis in childhood: Position paper of the European academy of allergology and clinical immunology. Allergy. 2007;**62**(8):857-871

[72] Sicherer SH, Simons FER. Self-injectable epinephrine for first-aid management of anaphylaxis. Pediatrics. 2007;**119**(3):638-646

[73] Noone HA, Novak-Wegrzyn S. Use of epinephrine in food – induced anaphylaxis. The Journal of Allergy and Clinical Immunology. 2007;**119**:S29-S100

[74] Kelso JM. A second dose of epinephrine for anaphylaxis: How often needed and how to carry. The Journal of Allergy and Clinical Immunology. 2006;**117**:464-465

[75] Oren E, Banerji A, Clark S, Camargo CA. Food- induced anaphylaxis and repeat epinephrine treatments. The Journal of Allergy and Clinical Immunology. 2007;**119**:S114

Section 4

Treatment

Chapter 6

Current Developments in Allergen-Specific Immunotherapy: A Brief Review

Mariana Giarola Benedito Bartholazzi, Tatiana de Morais Lodi and Olga Lima Tavares Machado

Abstract

Immunotherapy is a treatment for patients with type I-mediated allergic diseases. Molecular forms of allergen-specific immunotherapy (AIT), based on inducing immunological tolerance characterized by increased IL-10, TGF-β, and IgG4 levels, and Treg cell are continuously emerging to improve the efficacy of the treatment, shorten the duration of protocols, and prevent any side effects. This review covers the recent progress in AIT and routes of antigen administration. Classical immunotherapy uses allergen extracts obtained from natural sources. Limitations of the uses of these extracts, such as sensitizations with nonspecific agents, can be avoided using purified components, hypoallergenic recombinant proteins, and vaccines based on peptides (epitopes). However, these molecules have low immunogenicity requiring new carriers or more effective adjuvants. Vaccines based on carrier-bound B-cell epitope-containing peptides and the constructions of allergens coupled to virus-like particles (VLPs) are under evaluation. The possibility of vaccinating with DNA encoding the allergen to obtain an allergen-specific Th1 and IgG response is in development and the success of messenger ribonucleic acid (mRNA) vaccines against severe acute respiratory syndrome Coronavirus 2 must encourage as well the re-exploration of mRNA vaccine platform for innovative AIT.

Keywords: allergen-specific immunotherapy, vaccine, allergen, routes of administration, safety of immunotherapies

1. Introduction

Epigenetic factors and changes in the population's lifestyle are some of the factors that have contributed to the increase in IgE-mediated allergies worldwide. Data from the World Health Organization reveal that about 30% of the world population suffers from allergies in all age groups. Due to this increase and the effect that allergic diseases have on people's quality of life, a treatment, or even a cure, has been a priority among researchers, doctors, and society [1, 2]. Allergic reaction episodes are usually controlled with medication; however, the only treatment that acts on the immunological cause of the disease is allergen-specific immunotherapy (AIT) [2]. AIT is used to treat various forms of allergic diseases involving type I hypersensitivity, as it can modify TH2-driven immune responses by reducing symptoms after exposure to the allergen [3, 4].

Upon receiving a dose of immunotherapy containing the allergen, a shift from the allergenic TH2 inflammatory profile to the TH1 inflammatory profile and the generation of regulatory immune cells occurs. Decreased levels of mast cells, basophils, and eosinophils are seen in the mucosa and an increase in the production of allergen-specific regulatory T and B cells (Treg/Breg) occurs [5].

The generation of regulatory T cells (Treg) is the key event for the development of immune tolerance. Immune tolerance occurs in a peripheral and specific way, where the first is initiated by the secretion of IL-10 and TGF-β by allergen-specific Treg cells during continuous exposure and the second is associated with the increase in cells that present CD3+, CD25+ markers, and FOXP3+ in the nasal mucosa [6].

Essential features of AIT suggest that it has many advantages for the treatment of allergy because it works on a specific type of allergen and thus leads the individual's immune system to establish an immune response against the one who caused the disease [7, 8]. Furthermore, allergy vaccines can be produced relatively quickly and inexpensively compared to treatments with biological agents. Another advantage is that, unlike treatments with an anti-inflammatory profile, AIT can stop the progression of both mild allergy (rhinitis) and more severe forms such as asthma, modifying the natural course of the disease [9–11]. However, some aspects need to be considered for the success of immunotherapy. The first is that AIT is in the group of precision medicine treatments, where the allergens causing the disease need to be identified so that the correct vaccine is administered. The second aspect is the need to produce effective and safe vaccines against different allergens to be co-administered, thus causing polysensitization. Furthermore, thirdly, the administration of AIT can cause side effects in patients [12, 13].

Molecular allergy diagnostics (MA) is currently the most helpful patient selection method for prescribing allergen-specific immunotherapy (AIT). Component-resolved diagnosis (CRD) was established in 1980 as a new concept in allergy diagnosis. The CRD identifies a specific IgE toward natural or recombinant allergens rather than raw allergen extracts to determine a patient's sensitization at the molecular level [14]. More than 130 allergen molecules are commercialized. For more precise identification of the allergen, assays such as singleplex-ImmunoCAP, ImmuLite, and HyTech or many allergens per sample depot in microarrays (multiplex platform-ImmunoCAP ISAC-ThermoFisher Scientific/Phadia) can be employed [15, 16]. On the other hand, allergy Immunoproteomics can be an excellent ally for identifying unknown allergens. Proteomics has become critical to identify and structurally characterize allergens, including in vitro diagnostics, allergen discovery, and the analysis of biologicals proposed for AIT [11, 17].

Concerns about patient safety and treatment efficacy are the main reasons for the search for new approaches to AIT, so we have brought together several strategies that have been proposed to improve the effectiveness and safety of immunotherapies.

1.1 Technologies in the development of AIT—Molecular Approaches to AIT

The first to work with allergen-specific immunotherapy (AIT) was Noon [18], injecting grass pollen extracts into allergic patients. In this study, Noon was able to observe a reduction in symptoms and greater allergen tolerance for almost 1 year. Later, in 1935, Cooke and his team [19], after successful clinical trials, demonstrated that AIT induces allergen protection through specific IgG antibodies that can suppress allergen-induced skin inflammation.

Allergen-specific immunotherapies (AIT) use allergen extracts obtained from natural sources. Characteristically, the active products in AIT are a combination of allergens with other proteins extracted from biological sources (egg, pollen, and mites), used without alteration or treated with aldehydes, and then formulated with or without an adjuvant [5]. The new proposals to produce AIT rely on recombinant, synthetic proteins, or DNA, instead of using natural extracts of allergens in their formulation. After identifying the genomic sequence of interest or the allergen itself, these are extensively tested through in vitro assays and animal models to obtain information about their allergenicity and immunogenicity [20].

The molecular era of AIT employs native recombinants, hypoallergenic recombinants, peptides containing short, and nonreactive IgE T-cell epitopes, followed by hypoallergenic recombinant peptides, as AITs needed to improve immediately in two aspects: specificity and safety [21].

A summary of each of the molecular approaches currently used for AIT will be presented below.

1.1.1 Native recombinants

The use of native recombinants offers advantages over natural allergen extracts as they are well defined and contain relevant epitopes. Although, native recombinants cause immediate and late-phase side effects like natural allergens because of preserved IgE reactivity and T-cell epitopes. Thus, the preparation of AIT with these recombinants requires the maintenance of dosing schedules and multiple maintenance injections. However, the high quality of the vaccine (low cost and reproducibility) is the main advantage over natural extracts [22].

After producing the first recombinant allergens, it was demonstrated through in vitro experiments that the characteristics and the high proportion of epitopes resembled the allergen extracts [23]. Two other critical AIT studies also demonstrate this: in the survey by Jutel et al. [24], a mixture of 5 recombinant grass pollen demonstrated that a recombinant allergen vaccine can be an effective and safe treatment to improve the symptoms of allergic rhinitis. Clinical benefit is associated with modification of the specific immune response with IgG4 production and reduction of IgE antibodies consistent with the induction of IL-10-producing regulatory T cells. And the study by Pauli et al. [25] showed the efficacy of an AIT with native recombinants for the treatment of birch allergic rhinoconjunctivitis, concluding that the vaccine was safe and effective in the treatment of birch pollen allergy and induced a highly specific immune response.

1.1.2 Hypoallergenic recombinants

Recombinant hypoallergenic derivatives are characterized by having a reduced reactivity to IgE. Several techniques have been developed to reduce IgE reactivity, including fragmentation, oligomerization, mutation, and sequence reassembly [26]. Hypoallergens do not cause immediate side effects. However, after immunization, they induce specific IgG antibodies. Allergen-specific T-cell epitopes remain preserved in these molecules and may lead to late-phase T-cell mediated side effects [21].

In this sense, a clinical study with patients not allergic to birch pollen was carried out for 2 years. Three injections were administered subcutaneously with a monthly interval of a vaccine containing hypoallergenic recombinants obtained from the mentioned allergen. Vaccine administration also took place before the period of the first birch pollen season, with a booster dose later given before the next birch pollen season, thus allowing better monitoring of vaccination in the face of seasonal exposure to the allergen. It was observed that most patients immunized with the hypoallergenic recombinant vaccine induced levels of IgG antibodies against the allergen Bet v 1, which suggests that these antibodies act by blocking the IgE interaction with the allergen Bet v 1 [27].

Another model of recombinant hypoallergens is peptides containing transporter-linked B cell epitopes, where the presence of allergen-specific T cell epitopes is reduced to decrease allergen activity further, thus increasing safety. The use of carrier molecules on these peptides facilitates their production and increases their immunogenicity and ability to induce blocking IgG antibody responses [21, 28].

1.1.3 Carrier-bound B-cell epitope-containing peptides

A complement to hypoallergenic recombinants is the construction of peptides containing B cell epitopes linked to a transporter [28]. Vaccines containing B cell epitopes are composed of small peptides that cannot react with IgE, being obtained from allergens, specifically from the sites where the interaction with this antibody occurs. With the transporter, they offer patients a good IgG response that works by blocking the binding of the allergen to IgE [8].

These vaccines are produced from the fusion of recombinant proteins by expression in a bacterial system, using *Escherichia coli*, where the fused proteins are delivered in large quantities and quality [29]. Another essential characteristic of vaccines obtained from B cell epitopes is the reduction of their allergenic potential, since small fragments are used, which allows for the administration of higher doses, as well as their immunogenic potential, which makes it possible to administration of approximately three doses throughout the year, thus contributing to patient adherence to the treatment of allergic diseases [8].

BM32 is a B-cell epitope-based vaccine built to treat grass pollen allergy that has already been evaluated in several clinical trials and is the most advanced vaccine [30].

An important allergen from peanuts is Ara h 2. A fusion protein of the S-layer protein, SlpB from *Lactobacillus buchneri* CD034, and the Ara h 2-derived peptide AH3a42 was produced. This peptide comprised immunodominant B-cell epitopes as well as one T-cell epitope [31].

A study was carried out with Der p 1, a potent mite allergen responsible for causing respiratory allergies, for obtaining a fusion protein of a tetanus toxoid molecule with two copies of a peptide with hypoallergenic characteristics, previously identified through bioinformatics tools. After getting the protein DpTTDp, mice were immunized to assess the allergenic potential and production of IgG antibodies. It was observed in this study that the protein DpTTDp induced relevant levels of IgG antibodies, which act by inhibiting the interaction with IgE of patients allergic to mites, making it a candidate for a vaccine based on B cell epitope for the treatment of allergies to mites [32].

Another similar study was carried out with Salsola kali pollen, an allergen that triggers allergic rhinitis in dry and desert areas worldwide. A hypoallergenic vaccine based on B-cell epitopes was designed and called Sal k 1-KLH, composed of a peptide derived from the allergen Sal k 1 conjugated to the keyhole limpet hemocyanin transporter molecule. This study showed that the vaccine produced high IgG levels in immunized mice that block IgE interaction but did not show a T cell lymphocyte response compared to the extract and the recombinant [33].

1.1.4 Peptides containing T cell epitopes

Peptide-based immunotherapy (PIP) has been considered a safe strategy for epitope-based vaccines. Peptides must contain T cell epitopes. Peptides cannot bind IgE but bind to major histocompatibility complexes. Successful trials involve Japanese cedar pollen, grass pollens, ragweed, cat allergen Fel d 1 [34], honeybee venom, and house dust mite [35]. The role of innate immune cells in allergen immunotherapy that confers immune tolerance to the sensitizing allergen is unclear. The efficacy of immunotherapy is underscored by the induction of tolerance (T helper cell type 2 anergy Treg cell upregulation of immune deviation) and modification of innate and adaptive immune responses. It is speculated that they can induce [36].

Through epitope mapping studies, it is possible to identify which protein sequence is related to the induction of immunological tolerance and which does not participate in the inflammatory process triggered by the allergen. This is because peptides based on allergen epitopes have essential characteristics used in the clinical field to bind to a variety of class II HLA molecules [37].

An in silico study was carried out with the aeroallergen Zea M 1, a corn pollen allergen responsible for causing allergic reactions. The study aimed to evaluate the epitopes that had the potential to compose a vaccine based on the combination of B and T cell epitopes. After identifying B and T cell epitopes through prediction analyses, it was observed that the T cell epitope (AEWKPMPSW) presented an ideal and stable fit to the binding groove of the MHC I complex from B cells. The epitope KVPPPGPNITTNY remained conserved among homologous allergens and showed more significant potential for the vaccine [38]. The vaccine strategy based on T-cell epitopes is also being investigated for food allergies. First, the peptides were synthesized, and the T cell epitopes were mapped through assays of the proliferation of T cell responses in allergen-sensitized mice. Subsequently, the animals were treated with synthetic peptides and evaluated for antibody and cytokine levels. It was found in animals a reduction in symptoms and levels of cytokines and antibodies manifested in the allergic process, as well as a shift in response to a Th1 pattern and the production of IgG2a antibodies, which are characterized as adequate immunotherapy to treat allergy to shrimp [36, 39].

1.1.5 Allergens coupled to immunomodulatory compounds

Vaccines proposed a 100 years ago, and still used today, employ crude extracts and attenuated viruses. After identification of the allergens structures, AIT began to use recombinant proteins and epitope-peptides. However, highly refined antigens and derived peptides present low immunogenicity and often lead to the stimulation of weak and short-lived immunity, not activating all facets of the immune response, requiring adjustment of new immunostimulatory adjuvants to enhance immune responses induced by poorly immunogenic antigens. There are only a few adjuvants approved for human use. Alum, various aluminum salts, and the first and most commonly used adjuvant were the only human vaccine adjuvant for more than nine decades until 2009 [40]. Alum is not compatible with mucosal vaccines and is unsuitable for aluminum intolerant individuals. In 2009, the Food and Drug Administration (FDA) approved AS04, a combination of alum and monophosphoryl lipid A (MPLA), for human use [41]. From 2016 to 2018, the FDA approved three more adjuvants (i.e., MF59/AS03, CpG 1018, and AS01b). The first, MF59/AS03 is a squalene-based oil-in-water emulsion used in influenza vaccines [42]. The adjuvant CpG 1018 is a short synthetic oligonucleotide, agonist of TLR9 that is being used in a vaccine against hepatitis B. moreover, AS01b is a combined adjuvant containing MPLA and saponin QS-21 in a liposomal formulation that induces strong humoral immune responses and cellular and has been approved by the FDA for use in Shingrix® against herpes zoster and by the European Medicines Agency (EMA) for use in Mosquirix® against malaria [40].

Studies have found that CpG oligodeoxynucleotides are helpful as adjuvants in inducing Th1-type immune responses, demonstrating their immunomodulatory activity in a murine model of asthma, as they improve the function of antigen-presenting cells and increase the generation of vaccine-specific humoral and cellular immune responses [43]. Based on this technology, a randomized, double-blind, placebo-controlled, phase 2 trial of a vaccine based on ragweed pollen antigen (Amb 1), conjugated to an immunostimulatory DNA phosphorothioate oligodeoxyribonucleotide (AIC), was done in 25 adults allergic to the pollen of this plant. In this work, the vaccine (with a regimen of 6 weeks) offered long-term clinical efficacy in treating ragweed allergic rhinitis [44].

A powerful strategy for safe development of AIT is the covalent conjugation of allergens to toll-like receptor (TLR) agonists. Méndez et al. [45], synthesized two families of ligands, an 8-oxoadenine derivative as a ligand for TLR7 and a pyrimido[5,4-b]indole as a ligand for TLR4, both conjugated to a T-cell peptide from Pru p 3, one of major allergen from Prunus persica (Peach). These conjugates interacted with dendritic cells, inducing their specific maturation, T cell proliferation, and cytokine production in peach-allergic patients. In addition, they increased the frequencies of Treg cells in these patients and could induce IL-10 production [45].

1.1.6 Virus-like particle-coupled allergens

The construction of allergens coupled to virus-like particles (VLPs) started from a similar principle to that described for allergens coupled to immunomodulatory sequences. In this technique, the allergen molecules are chemically coupled or specific binding systems to virus-like particles through recombinant expression [46]. This technology has shown reduced allergenic activity in vaccines and good immunogenicity. The impediment to its use, on the other hand, is the difficulty in producing the vaccines in a replicable way due to the uncontrollable coupling process [21]. A sophisticated approach to engineering virus-like nanoparticles (VNPs) has been demonstrated by Kueng et al. [47]. This work showed that the cDNA encoding the allergen was coupled to the DNA encoding the virus.

In a preclinical trial of allergy to mugwort pollen (also known as a queen of grass, field chamomile, or fireweed), these particles were used successfully for prophylactic vaccination [48]. Virus-like particles (VLPs) are safe platforms for inducing protective antibodies, and several VLP-based vaccines are commercially available, including cat allergens. In a previous study, a vaccine composed of Qβ-derived VLPs coupled to the cat allergen Fel d 1 was highly immunogenic and capable of inducing IgG antibodies in mice. Immunization of Fel d 1 sensitized mice with protected Qβ-Fel d 1 against anaphylaxis after challenge with Fel d 1 allergen [49]. A recent study showed that the allergens displayed in Qβ-VLP are immunogenic but not reactogenic and do not activate human mast cells. VLP could constitute a platform to deliver allergens to allergic patients immunogenically and effectively but safely. Storni et al. [50] tested peanut allergy vaccine candidates based on the immunologically optimized VLP derived from cucumber mosaic virus (CuMVtt). They demonstrated that the inactivated, VLP-coupled allergen reduced systemic and local allergic symptoms after challenge with the whole allergen extract (composed of about 12 allergenic proteins), demonstrating that immunization against a single allergen protected against a mixture of allergens could be a hope for patients allergic to many components of an extract from a single source [50].

1.1.7 Nucleic acids encoding allergens

Publications from three decades ago showed that nucleic acid constructs (plasmid DNA or mRNA) could be injected into mice, resulting in the encoded protein made in situ. An initial study demonstrated that plasmid DNA encoding virus antigens could result in the generation of immune responses, so efforts were directed toward the use of plasmid DNA in vaccines [51].

Nucleotide vaccines are vectors that encode antigens and retain adjuvant-like activity by stimulating innate immune responses that contribute to adaptive responses [52]. Some questions were raised on whether a DNA vaccine could initiate an autoimmune disease since anti-DNA antibodies are a hallmark of autoimmune diseases. The results demonstrate that there is safety in using these vaccines and that this incorporation does not occur [51].

DNA vaccination presents the ability to rapidly induce strong CD4 and CD8 T cell and antibody responses. Several animal models for allergic diseases have demonstrated that DNA vaccination can induce a Th1 type immune response, which could counterbalance the Th2 response. Immunomic Therapeutics, Inc.'s research group developed novel allergy immunotherapy based on LAMP technology to treat pollen-induced allergies. Lysosomal Associated Membrane Protein 1 (LAMP-1 or LAMP) is a lysosomal residential protein. It has been shown that the inclusion of LAMP in the DNA plasmids significantly enhanced both cellular and humoral responses in vaccinated animals. The LAMP-Vax platform utilizes an up-to-date targeting approach, which should avoid therapy-induced side effects caused by high amounts of free allergen. Alternatively, the synthesized allergen-LAMP fusion protein is directly shuttled into the lysosomal compartment, circumventing the patient's exposure to the native allergen. Instead of inducing tolerance, this therapy is designed to reverse the allergenic IgE/TH2 response toward an IgG/TH1 response [53].

Cry j 1 and Cry j 2 proteins are the 2 major allergenic components in Japanese red cedar (JRC) pollen and cause pollinosis (JCP) in 30–35% of the Japanese population. Su et al. [54] demonstrated that DNA plasmids encoding LAMP fused with Cry j 1 and Cry j 2 proteins elicited a strong Th1 response in mice. After repeated allergen exposure, vaccinated mice were well protected, as indicated by a minimal level of allergen-specific IgE production. The safety and immunological effects of an investigational DNA vaccine encoding CryJ2-LAMP were evaluated by Phase IA and IB clinical trials. Results indicated that CryJ2-LAMP DNA vaccine is safe and has the potential therapeutic potential for JRC and/or Mountain Cedar (MC) sensitive subjects.

Studies in Phase 1 trials to evaluate the safety, tolerability, and immune response in adolescents or adults allergic to peanut allergens employing multivalent peanut-LAMP-1 DNA vaccine, including Ara h 1, Ara h 2, and Ara h 3, are promising [55].

1.1.8 IgG blocking antibodies specific to recombinant allergens

To obtain vaccines defined for passive immunization, specific blocking antibodies for human allergens are necessary. The first published studies where these allergen-specific antibodies were reported appeared more than two decades ago [21]. A combinatorial library to obtain IgE was constructed from peripheral blood mononuclear cells of an allergic patient to grass pollen where, for the first time, the Fabs regions of IgE specific for human allergens were isolated [56]. An IgE Fab specific for the major grass pollen allergen (Phl p 2) was converted into recombinant human IgG, and this blocked the Phl p 2 induced basophil degranulation, thus demonstrating its therapeutic potential [57].

Bi-specific antibodies were created so that an IgG-specific recombinant allergen could block the entry of allergens through the respiratory epithelium. It was possible to demonstrate the immobilization of allergen-specific IgG blocking antibodies using IgG specific for ICAM1 in respiratory epithelial cells, thus preventing the entry of allergens and opening up possibilities for topical treatment using blocking antibodies [58]. The idea of passive immunization from allergen-specific recombinant IgG antibodies is exciting and is undoubtedly a possible approach for allergen sources that contain mainly a significant allergen that can be blocked with one or a few monoclonal antibodies. This approach will be beneficial for seasonal allergies, as a pre-seasonal immunization can effectively protect the patient during seasonal exposure to the allergen [21].

1.1.9 Cell-based therapy

This technology for formulating a safer immunotherapy is based on the classic studies of hematopoietic stem cell transfer from one mouse strain to another strain with different MHC origins early in life [21]. From that study, Baranyi et al., [59] demonstrated that rats received such cells that express the allergen could not be sensitized against the corresponding allergen. Furthermore, even using a sensitization protocol with aluminum hydroxide adsorbed allergens, it was not possible to induce allergen-specific T cells, antibodies (of any isotype, including IgE), or allergic immune responses, indicating that a robust lifetime tolerance was achieved, which depend on mechanisms of central tolerance rather than peripheral regulation.

This technique has an immunomodulatory treatment, uses a protocol for cell transduction – which can be dangerous – and needs to be applied early in life, probably immediately after birth. However, a cell-based treatment shows that a robust, lifelong, allergen-specific immune tolerance is achievable [21].

The cell-based allergen-specific prevention approach is highly experimental, warranting further investigation in clinical trials, as major safety hurdles can be overcome [21].

2. Routes of administration

Other approaches are being sought to try to reduce the risks of side effects and have a safer AIT and with that alternative routes of administration have been studied.

Subcutaneous immunotherapy (SCIT) is the route of administration with the most well-established underlying mechanisms and has been in use since 1911. Already the Sublingual immunotherapy (SLIT) has been considered due to its ease of use and reduced side effects [21].

The appropriate candidates for AIT are mainly children with allergic asthma. The use of molecular diagnosis techniques [component-resolved diagnostics (CRD)] increases the effectiveness of AIT since it allows physicians to identify better whether children with allergic respiratory symptoms are sensitized to major allergens or cross-reactive molecules [60].

A review by Tsaburi [61] and colleagues gives us an understanding of the use of SCIT and SLIT in the treatment of children with allergic asthma. Studies have shown a significant decrease in asthma symptoms and also a preventive effect at the onset of the disease. And while SLIT safety profile appears better, some results suggest that SCIT efficacy is better with an earlier onset than SLIT in children with allergic asthma. Furthermore, there is no effective SLIT for significant allergens such as food and aeroallergens [62, 63].

Another approach to improving AIT is oral immunotherapy (OIT). This pathway has been tested primarily for allergens from food sources that are resistant to digestion, such as milk, egg, peanuts, and wheat, while not being used for other allergen sources [21].

Clinical studies show that the advantages of OIT are associated with the induction of specific IgG antibodies, which can block the IgE-allergen interaction as well as in SCIT. It was also described that oral immunotherapy induced changes in cellular immune responses, which could lead to clinical oral tolerance [64].

Intralymphatic Immunotherapy (ILIT) is a new application approach that has been developed within subcutaneous immunotherapy (SCIT). The proposal for this route of administration is the large amount of immune system cells that lymph nodes present, and a direct exposure of the allergen to these cells will induce a protective IgG response and faster immunomodulation [65].

A recent review by Senti et al. [66] provides an excellent overview about intralymphatic AIT, ultrasound-guided injection of allergen extracts into lymph nodes. However, there are no studies comparing the immunological and clinical responses of ILIT and SCIT using vaccines of the same allergen, making it difficult to confirm whether intralymphatic immunotherapy induces faster and stronger responses than subcutaneous.

ILIT has an acceptable safety profile, but its disadvantage is the need to use an ultrasound device for vaccine application in lymph nodes. Furthermore, few studies have been carried out so far when compared to other routes [67].

Epicutaneous immunotherapy (EPIT) assumed that applying allergens through the non-vascularized epidermis would induce fewer systemic side effects [21].

Another critical point is that EPIT does not use a needle, being considered especially suitable for children. Furthermore, this type of immunotherapy uses high doses of allergen and, despite showing some improvement in seasonal symptoms, it does not show considerable benefit in terms of local side effects when compared to subcutaneous immunotherapy (SCIT) [68].

Routes for administration	Advantages	Disadvantage	References
SCIT—subcutaneous injection	Best mechanisms documented applicable for most allergen sources	Severe side effects rares but possible; Injection needed	[18, 61, 63]
SLIT—sublingual application in form of drops or tablets under the tongue by self-administration	Clinical efficacy demonstrated in studies	Less effective than SCIT Mechanisms are less well defined than for SCIT cumbersome treatment with low compliance applicable / available only for few allergen sources	[61, 62]
OIT—Oral administration and swallowing	Effective for food allergey	High rate of side effects	[64]
ILIT—Ultrasound-guided injection into subcutaneous lymphnodes	Experimental AIT form Clinical efficacy partly shown	Ultrasound-guided injection needed Advantage over SCIT not demonstrated	[65–67]
EPIT—epicutaneous administration on stripped skin	Experimental AIT form	Clinical efficacy not demonstrated	[68]

Table 1.
Routes for administration of AIT, showing the advantages and disadvantages of each route.

Table 1 brings together all the proposed administration routes, showing the advantages and disadvantages that each one presents.

3. Conclusion

Allergen-specific immunotherapy has been applied for over a 100 years. This review emphasized the fundamental importance of accurately identifying the structure of allergens and their dominant epitopes, as well as choosing adjuvants. For the market establishment or acceptance new molecular AIT preparations would be the demonstration of clear added value, e.g., shortened therapy duration and superior effectiveness or tolerability. Despite the development of new approaches to allergen-specific immunotherapy, licensing any vaccine for the clinic proved complicated. Currently, allergen-specific immunotherapy with extracts of natural allergens is the only universally approved treatment for allergic patients. Isolated treatments are made with purified allergens to avoid adverse effects caused by the allergenicity of natural extracts. The latest generation of allergy vaccines based on T-cell epitopes and B-cell epitopes linked to carriers has the potential to transform AIT as it can prevent side effects, allowing the administration of doses to induce strong allergen-specific IgG responses and provide patients with sensitized with lasting effects.

AIT, like other therapies, has advantages and disadvantages in its use, but with new technologies and molecular strategies much has been sought so that safer AIT is developed and better routes of administration are developed, revolutionizing traditional immunotherapy-based in natural allergenic strata. Since success of COVID-19 vaccine allergen DNA and mRNA vaccination has been gaining prominence.

We hope that more people will benefit from this preventive way of controlling allergic diseases.

Abbreviations

AIT	Allergen-specific immunotherapy
CRD	Component-resolved diagnosis
EPIT	Epicutaneous immunotherapy
FDA	Food and Drug Administration
ILIT	Intralymphatic Immunotherapy
LAMP	Lysosomal Associated Membrane Protein
LTP	Transfer protein of lipids
MA	Molecular allergy diagnostics
MPLA	Monophosphoryl lipid A
OIT	Oral immunotherapy
PIP	Peptide-based immunotherapy
SCIT	Subcutaneous immunotherapy
SLIT	Sublingual immunotherapy
TLR	Toll-like receptor
VLPs	Virus-like particles

Author details

Mariana Giarola Benedito Bartholazzi, Tatiana de Morais Lodi and Olga Lima Tavares Machado*
Universidade Estadual do Norte Fluminense -Darcy Ribeiro, Centro de Biociências e Biotecnologia, Rio de Janeiro, Brasil

*Address all correspondence to: olgauenf@yahoo.com.br

References

[1] Stefan S, Kirsten K, Sonja W, Nadine D, Andrea W, Andreas R, et al. Conjugation of wildtype and hypoallergenic mugwort allergen Art v 1 to flagellin induces IL-10-DC and suppresses allergen-specific TH2-responses in vivo. Scientific Reports. 2017;**7**:1-16. DOI: 10.1038/s41598-017-11972-w

[2] Jongejan L, Van RR, Poulsen LK, Van RR. Immunotherapy hypoallergenic molecules for subcutaneous immunotherapy. Expert Review of Clinical Immunology. 2016;**12**:5-7. DOI: org/10.1586/1744666X.2016.1103182

[3] Frew AJ. Immunotherapy of allergic disease. In: Clinical Immunology eBook; Fifth ed. Elsevier. 2019. pp. 1227-1235 ISBN: 9780702070396

[4] James C, Bernstein DI. Allergen immunotherapy: An updated review of safety. Current Opinion in Allergy and Clinical Immunology. 2017;**17**:55-59

[5] Shamji MH, Durham SR. Mechanisms of allergic diseases mechanisms of allergen immunotherapy for inhaled allergens and predictive biomarkers. The Journal of Allergy and Clinical Immunology. 2017;**140**:1485-1498. DOI: 10.1016/j.jaci.2017.10.010

[6] Sackesen C, Van De VW, Akdis M, Soyer O, Zumkehr J, Ruckert B, et al. Suppression of B-cell activation and IgE, IgA, IgG1 and IgG4 production by mammalian telomeric oligonucleotides. Allergy. 2013;**68**:593-603. DOI: 10.1111/all.12133

[7] Jutel M, Agache I, Bonini S, Burks AW, Calderon M, Canonica W, et al. International consensus on allergy immunotherapy. The Journal of Allergy and Clinical Immunology. 2015;**136**:556-568. DOI: 10.1016/j.jaci.2015.04.047

[8] Valenta R, Campana R, Focke-Tejkl M, Niederberger V. Vaccine development for allergen-specific immunotherapy based on recombinant allergens and synthetic allergen peptides: Lessons from the past and novel mechanisms of action for the future. The Journal of Allergy and Clinical Immunology. 2016;**137**:351-357. DOI: 10.1016/j.jaci.2015.12.1299

[9] Jacobsen L, Niggemann B, Dreborg S, Ferdousi HA, Halken S, Koivikko A, et al. Original article specific immunotherapy has long-term preventive effect of seasonal and perennial asthma: 10-year follow-up on the PAT study. 2007. Allergy. 2007;**62**(943-8). DOI: 10.1111/j.1398-9995.2007.01451.x

[10] Valovirta E. Effect of AIT in children including potential to prevent the development of asthma. Allergy. 2011;**66**:53-54. DOI: 10.1111/j.1398-9995.2011.02640.x

[11] Pav GF, Parra-vargas MI, Ram F, Melgoza-ruiz E, Serrano-p NH, Teran LM. Allergen immunotherapy: Current and future trends. Cell. 2022;**11**:212-234. DOI: 10.3390/cells11020212

[12] Valenta R, Karaulov A, Niederberger V, Gattinger P, van Hage M, Flicker S, et al. Molecular aspects of allergens and allergy. Advances in Immunology. 2018;**138**:195-256. DOI: 10.1016/bs.ai.2018.03.002

[13] Zhernov Y, Curin M, Khaitov M, Karaulov A, Valenta R. Recombinant allergens for immunotherapy. Current Opinion in Allergy and Clinical

Immunology. 2019;**19**:402-414. DOI: 10.1097/ACI.0000000000000536

[14] Sastre J, Sastre-ibañez M. Molecular diagnosis and immunotherapy. Current Opinion in Allergy and Clinical Immunology. 2016;**16**:565-570

[15] Koch L, Laipold K, Arzt-Gradwohl L, Čerpes U, Sturm EM, Aberer W, et al. IgE multiplex testing in house dust mite allergy is utile and sensitivity is comparable to extract-based singleplex testing. Allergy. 2020;**75**:2091-2094. DOI: 10.1111/all.14271

[16] Matricardi PM, Hoffmann HJ, Valenta R, Hilger C, Hofmaier S, Aalberse RC, et al. EAACI Molecular Allergology User ' s Guide. Pediatr Allergy Immunology. 2016. Suppl 23:1-250. DOI: 10.1111/pai.12563

[17] Morales-amparano MB, Valenzuela-corral A, Escobedo-moratilla A, Montfort GR, Luz V, Teran LM, et al. Immunoproteomic identification of allergenic proteins in pecan (Carya illinoinensis) pollen. Journal of Proteomics. 2021;**248**:e104348. DOI: 10.1016/j.jprot.2021.104348

[18] Noon L. Prophylactic inoculation against hay fever. 1911. International Archives of Allergy and Applied Immunology. 1953;**4**(4):285-288. DOI: 10.1159/000228032;1572-3

[19] Cooke RA, Barnard JH, Hebald S, Stull A. Serological evidence of immunity with coexisting sensitization in a type of human allergy (hay fever)*. The Journal of Experimental Medicine. 1935;**30**(62):733-750. DOI: 10.1084/jem.62.6.733

[20] Pfaar O, Agache I, Blay F, Bonini S, Durham MC, Gawlik R, et al. Perspectives in allergen immunotherapy: 2019 and beyond. The Journal of Experimental Medicine. 2019;**74**(108):3-25

[21] Dorofeeva Y, Shilovskiy I, Tulaeva I, Focke-tejkl M, Flicker S, Kudlay D, et al. Past, present , and future of allergen immunotherapy vaccines. Allergy. 2021;**76**:131-149. DOI: 10.1111/all.14300

[22] Isabel Tabar A, Prieto L, Alba P, Nieto A, Rodriguez M, Torrecillas M, et al. Double-blind, randomized, placebo-controlled trial of allergen-specific immunotherapy with the major allergen. Journal of Allergy Clinical Immunology. 2021;**144**:216-223

[23] Niederberger V, Laffer S, Fröschl R, Kraft D, Rumpold H, Kapiotis S, et al. IgE antibodies to recombinant pollen allergens (Phl p 1, Phl p 2, Philp p 5, and Bet v 2) account for a high percentage of grass pollen-specific IgE. The Journal of Allergy and Clinical Immunology. 1998;**101**:258-264. DOI: 10.1016/s0091-6749(98)70391-4

[24] Jutel M, Jaeger L, Suck R, Meyer H, Fiebig H, Cromwell O. Allergen-specific immunotherapy with recombinant grass pollen allergens. The Journal of Allergy and Clinical Immunology. 2005;**116**:608-613. DOI: 10.1016/j.jaci.2005.06.004

[25] Pauli G, Larsen TH, Rak S, Horak F, Pastorello E, Valenta R, et al. Efficacy of recombinant birch pollen vaccine for the treatment of birch-allergic rhinoconjunctivitis. The Journal of Allergy and Clinical Immunology. 2008;**122**:951-960. DOI: 10.1016/j.jaci.2008.09.017

[26] Spertini F, Perrin Y, Audran R, Pellaton C, Boudousquié C, Barbier N, et al. Safety and immunogenicity of immunotherapy with Bet v 1-derived contiguous overlapping peptides. The Journal of Allergy and Clinical

Immunology. 2014;**134**:239-240.e13. DOI: 10.1016/j.jaci.2014.04.001

[27] Campana R, Marth K, Zieglmayer P, Weber M, Lupinek C, Zhernov Y, et al. Vaccination of nonallergic individuals with recombinant hypoallergenic fragments of birch pollen allergen Bet v 1: Safety, effects, and mechanisms. Journal of Allergy and Clinical Immunology. 2019;**143**:1258-1261. DOI: 10.1016/j.jaci.2018.11.011

[28] Zieglmayer P, Focke-Tejkl M, Schmutz R, Lemell P, Zieglmayer R, Weber M, et al. Mechanisms, safety and efficacy of a B cell epitope-based vaccine for immunotherapy of grass pollen allergy. eBioMedicine. 2016;**11**:43-57. DOI: 10.1016/j.ebiom.2016.08.022

[29] Niespodziana K, Focke-Tejkl M, Linhart B, Civaj V, Blatt K, Valent P, et al. A hypoallergenic cat vaccine based on Fel d 1-derived peptides fused to hepatitis B PreS. The Journal of Allergy and Clinical Immunology. 2011;**127**:1562-1570. DOI: 10.1016/j.jaci.2011.02.004

[30] Focke-Tejkl M, Weber M, Niespodziana K, Neubauer A, Huber H, Henning R, et al. Development and characterization of a recombinant, hypoallergenic, peptide-based vaccine for grass pollen allergy. The Journal of Allergy and Clinical Immunology. 2015;**1**(135):1207-1217. DOI: 10.1016/j.jaci.2014.09.012

[31] Anzengruber J, Bublin M, Bönisch E, Janesch B, Tscheppe A, Braun ML, et al. Lactobacillus buchneri S-layer as carrier for an Ara h 2-derived peptide for peanut allergen-specific immunotherapy. Molecular Immunology. 2017;**85**:81-88. DOI: 10.1016/j.molimm.2017.02.005

[32] Fanuel S, Tabesh S, Mokhtarian K, Saroddiny E. Construction of a recombinant B-cell epitope vaccine based on a Der p 1 -derived hypoallergen : A bioinformatics approach. Immunotherapy. 2018;**10**:537-553. DOI: 10.2217/imt-2017-0163

[33] Tabesh S, Fanuel S, Reza M, Saeed M. International immunopharmacology design and evaluation of a hypoallergenic peptide-based vaccine for Salsola kali allergy. International Immunopharmacology. 2019;**66**:62-68. DOI: 10.1016/j.intimp.2018.10.037

[34] Worm M, Lee H, Kleine-Tebb J, Hafner RP, Laidler P, Healey D, et al. Development and preliminary clinical evaluation of a peptide immunotherapy vaccine for cat allergy. The Journal of Allergy and Clinical Immunology. 2011;**127**:89-97. DOI: 10.1016/j.jaci.2010.11.029

[35] Ramchandani R, Hossenbaccus L, Ellis AK. Immunoregulatory T cell epitope peptides for the treatment of allergic disease. Immunotherapy. 2021;**15**:1283-1291. DOI: 10.2217/imt-2021-0133

[36] Xu LL, Lin H, Yu C, Zhao JL, Dang XW, Li ZX. Identi fi cation of the dominant T-cell epitopes of lit v 1 shrimp major allergen and their functional overlap with known B-cell epitopes. Journal of Agricultural and Food Chemistry. 2021;**69**:7420-7428. DOI: 10.1021/acs.jafc.1c02231

[37] O'Hehir RE, Prickett SR, Rolland JM, Rolland JM. T cell epitope peptide therapy for allergic diseases. Current Allergy and Asthma Reports. 2016;**16**:1-9. DOI: 10.1007/s11882-015-0587-0

[38] Basu A, Sarkar A, Basak P. Immunoinformatics based vaccine design for Zea M 1 Pollen Allergen. Journal of Young Pharmacists. 2018;**10**:260-266. DOI: 10.5530/jyp

[39] Wai CYY, Leung NYH, Leung PSC, Chu KH. T cell epitope immunotherapy ameliorates allergic responses in a murine model of shrimp allergy. Allergy. 2018;**46**:491

[40] Wang P. Natural and synthetic saponins as vaccine adjuvants. Vaccines (Basel). 2021;**9**:222. DOI: 10.3390/vaccines9030222

[41] Garçon N, Di Pasquale A. From discovery to licensure, the Adjuvant System story. Hum Vaccin Immunother. 2017;**13**:19-33. DOI: 10.1080/21645515.2016.1225635

[42] Cohet C, Van Der MR, Bauchau V, Bekkat-berkani R, Doherty TM, Schuind A, et al. Safety of AS03-adjuvanted influenza vaccines: A review of the evidence. Vaccine. 2019;**37**:3006-3021. DOI: 10.1016/j.vaccine.2019.04.048

[43] Banerjee B, Kelly KJ, Fink JN, Henderson JD, Bansal NK, Kurup VP. Modulation of airway inflammation by immunostimulatory CpG oligodeoxynucleotides in a murine model of allergic aspergillosis. Infection and Immunity. 2004;**72**:6087-6094. DOI: 10.1128/IAI.72.10.6087-6094.2004

[44] CreticosPS,SchroederJT,HamiltonRG, Balcer-Whaley SL, Khattignavong AP, Lindblad R, et al. Immunotherapy with a ragweed–toll-like receptor 9 agonist vaccine for allergic rhinitis. New England Journal of Medicine. 2006;**355**:1445-1455. DOI: 10.1056/NEJMoa052916

[45] Méndez JL, Palomares F, Gómez F, Ramírez-López P, Ramos-Soriano J, Torres MJ, et al. Immunomodulatory response of toll-like receptor ligand – peptide conjugates in food allergy. ACS Chemical Biology. 2021;**16**:2651-2664. DOI: 10.1021/acschembio.1c00765

[46] Engeroff P, Caviezel F, Storni F, Thoms F, Vogel M, Bachmann MF. Allergens displayed on virus-like particles are highly immunogenic but fail to activate human mast cells. European Journal of Allergy. 2021;**73**:341-349

[47] Kueng HJ, Manta C, Haiderer D, Leb VM, Schmetterer KG, Neunkirchner A, et al. Fluorosomes: A convenient new reagent to detect and block multivalent and complex receptor-ligand interactions. The FASEB Journal. 2010;**24**:1572-1582. DOI: 10.1096/fj.09-137281

[48] Kratzer B, Köhler C, Hofer S, Smole U, Trapin D, Iturri J, et al. Prevention of allergy by virus-like nanoparticles (VNP) delivering shielded versions of major allergens in a humanized murine allergy model. European Journal of Allergy. 2019;**74**:246-260. DOI: 10.1111/all.13573

[49] Schmitz N, Dietmeier K, Bauer M, Maudrich M, Utzinger S, Muntwiler S, et al. Displaying Fel d1 on virus-like particles prevents reactogenicity despite greatly enhanced immunogenicity: A novel therapy for cat allergy. Journal of Experimental Medicine. 2009;**206**: 1941-1955. DOI: 10.1084/ jem.20090199

[50] Storni F, Zeltins A, Balke I, Heath MD, Kramer MF. Vaccine against peanut allergy based on engineered virus-like particles displaying single major peanut allergens. Vaccine against peanut allergy based on engineered virus-like particles displaying single major peanut allergens. The Journal of Allergy and Clinical Immunology. 2020;**145**:1240-1253.e3. DOI: 10.1016/j.jaci.2019.12.007

[51] Fomsgaard A, Liu MA. The key role of nucleic acid vaccines for one health.

Viruses. 2021;**13**:258. DOI: 10.3390/v13020258

[52] Sharma A, Gaur P, BhuyanPawar S. Vaccine Development Based on Whole Cell Vaccine and Subunit Candidates by Using Proteomic and Genomic Assays. In: Vaccines & Vaccine Technologies. OMICS Group EBooks; 2014. pp. 1-14

[53] Scheiblhofer S, Thalhamer J, Weiss R. DNA and mRNA vaccination against allergies. Pediatric Allergy and Immunology. 2018;**29**:679-668. DOI: 10.1111/pai.12964

[54] Su Y, Romeu-bonilla E, Anagnostou A, Fitz-patrick D, Hearl W, Heiland T. Safety and long-term immunological effects of CryJ2- LAMP plasmid vaccine in Japanese red cedar atopic subjects: A phase I study. Human Vaccines & Immunotherapeutics. 2017;**13**:2804-2813. DOI: 10.1080/ 21645515.2017.1329070

[55] Astellas Pharma Global Development I. A study to evaluate safety tolerability and immune response in adolescents allergic to Peanut after receiving intradermal administration of ASP0892 (ARA-LAMP-vax) a single multivalent Peanut (Ara h1 h2 h3) lysosomal associated membrane protein DNA Plasmid 2022

[56] Steinberger P, Kraft D, Valenta R. Construction of a combinatorial IgE library from an allergic patient: Isolation and characterization of human IgE fabs with specificity for the major timothy grass pollen allergen, Phi p 5. The Journal of Biological Chemistry. 1996;**271**:10967-10972. DOI: 10.1074/jbc.271.18.10967

[57] Flicker S, Steinberger P, Norderhaug L, Sperr WR, Majlesi Y, Valent P, et al. Conversion of grass pollen allergen-specific human IgE into a protective IgG 1 antibody. European Journal of Immunology. 2002;**32**:2156-2162. DOI: 10.1002/1521-4141

[58] Madritsch C, Eckl-Dorna J, Blatt K, Ellinger I, Kundi M, Niederberger V, et al. Antibody conjugates bispecific for intercellular adhesion molecule 1 and allergen prevent migration of allergens through respiratory epithelial cell layers. The Journal of Allergy and Clinical Immunology. 2015;**136**:490-493. DOI: 10.1016/j.jaci.2015.01.006

[59] Baranyi U, Linhart B, Pilat N, Gattringer M, Bagley J, Muehlbacher F, et al. Tolerization of a Type I allergic immune response through transplantation of genetically modified hematopoietic stem cells. Journal of Immunology. 2015;**180**:8168-8175

[60] Canonica GW, Ansotegui IJ, Pawankar R, Schmid-Grendelmeier P, Van Hage M, Baena-Cagnani CE, et al. A WAO-ARIA-GA2LEN consensus document on molecular-based allergy diagnostics. World Allergy Organization Journal. 2013;**6**:1-17. DOI: 10.1186/1939-4551-6-17

[61] Tsabouri S, Mavroudi A, Feketea G, Guibas GV. Subcutaneous and sublingual immunotherapy in allergic asthma in children. Frontiers in Pediatrics. 2017;**21**(5):82. DOI: 10.3389/fped.2017.00082

[62] Durham SR, Yang WH, Pedersen MR, Johansen N, Rak S. Sublingual immunotherapy with once-daily grass allergen tablets: A randomized controlled trial in seasonal allergic rhinoconjunctivitis. The Journal of Allergy and Clinical Immunology. 2006;**117**:802-809. DOI: 10.1016/j.jaci.2005.12.1358

[63] Passalacqua G, Bagnasco D, Canonica GW. 30 years of sublingual immunotherapy. Allergy. 2020;**75**:1107-1120. DOI: 10.1111/all.14113

[64] Eiwegger T, Anagnostou K, Arasi S, Bégin P, Ben-Shoshan M, Beyer K, et al. Conflicting verdicts on peanut oral immunotherapy from the Institute for Clinical and Economic Review and US Food and Drug Administration Advisory Committee: Where do we go from here? The Journal of Allergy and Clinical Immunology. 2020;**145**:1153-1156. DOI: 10.1016/j.jaci.2019.10.021

[65] SentiG,PrinzVavrickaBM,ErdmannI, Diaz MI, Markus R, Mccormack SJ, et al. Intralymphatic allergen administration renders specific immunotherapy faster and safer: A randomized controlled trial. 2008. Proceedings of the National Academy of Sciences of the United States of America. 2008;**105**:17908-17912. DOI: 10.1073/pnas.0803725105

[66] Senti G, Freiburghaus U, Larenas-linnemann D, Jürgen H. Intralymphatic immunotherapy : Update and unmet needs. 2019. International Archives of Allergy and Immunology. 2019;**178**:141-149. DOI: 10.1159/000493647-9

[67] Senti G, Crameri R, Kuster D, Johansen P, Martinez-Gomez JM, Graf N, et al. Intralymphatic immunotherapy for cat allergy induces tolerance after only 3 injections. The Journal of Allergy and Clinical Immunology. 2012;**129**:1290-1296. DOI: 10.1016/j.jaci.2012.02.026

[68] Senti G, Von Moos S, Tay F, Graf N, Johansen P, Kündig TM. Determinants of efficacy and safety in epicutaneous allergen immunotherapy: Summary of three clinical trials. European Journal of Allergy. 2015;**70**:707-710. DOI: 10.1111/all.12600

Chapter 7

Mesenchymal Stem/Stromal Cells in Allergic Disease Management

Leisheng Zhang, Zhongchao Han and Xiaowei Gao

Abstract

Allergic diseases are a clump of disorders caused by protective or harmful immune responses to specific exogenous stimulations. To date, the worldwide prevalence of allergic diseases has caused considerable perplex to patients and guardians physically and mentally. Despite the significant advances in preclinical investigation and clinical practice, yet the effective treatment strategies for allergic diseases are far from satisfaction. State-of-the-art renewal has highlighted the involvement of mesenchymal stem/stromal cell (MSC)-based cytotherapy for various allergic disease management including atopic dermatitis, pediatric asthma, allergic rhinitis, and urticaria, which largely attributes to the unique immunomodulatory properties and mode of action via autocrine and paracrine, direct- or trans-differentiation. In this chapter, we mainly focus on the latest updates of MSC-based investigations upon allergic disease administration as well as the concomitant prospective and challenges, which will provide overwhelming new references for MSC-based cytotherapy in regenerative medicine.

Keywords: mesenchymal stem/stromal cells, allergic diseases, exosome, immunomodulation, allergic rhinitis, cytotherapy

1. Introduction

Allergic diseases, including atopic dermatitis, pediatric asthma, allergic rhinitis, and urticaria, have been recognized as one of the most prevalent chronic diseases and affected more than 300 million individuals all over the world and thus, have garnered public health attention worldwide over the past decades [1]. To date, a variety of factors (e.g., IL-6, IL-8, IL-25, IL-33, INF-γ) and noxious stimuli (e.g., microbiota, helminths, human milk immunological composition) in the environment have been involved in the occurrence or progression of allergic diseases [2, 3]. Of note, immunomodulation has been acknowledged as the core strategy for allergic and autoimmune diseases.

Despite the diversity in the pathogenic mechanism of governing the progression, a variety of key elements involved in allergic diseases have been identified such as immune cells (e.g., mast cells, T cells), antibodies, cytokines, epigenetic and genetic determinants [1, 4, 5]. For instance, of the aforementioned pathogenic factors, mast cells with inflammatory mediator expression have been recognized playing a key role in various allergic reactions and autoimmune processes [6, 7].

For decades, integrated prevention and intervention strategies have been developed for the remission of allergic diseases. For example, the European Academy of Allergy and Clinical Immunology (EAACI) guidelines for allergen immunotherapy (AIT) have been reported in preparations for the administration of allergic disease by Dhami and colleagues [8]. Meanwhile, JAK/STAT inhibitors, together with relevant small-molecule cytokine antagonists such as CRTH2 inhibitors and PDE4 inhibitors, have been tested in a spectrum of allergic diseases [9]. Additionally, current advances have also suggested the probiotics and prebiotics in the treatment or prevention of allergic diseases during the prenatal period [10–12]. For example, Tang et al. reviewed that prebiotic-supplemented formulas might be an effective alternative for preventing atopic eczema in infants with high probability of developing allergic disease [10, 13].

2. The overview of MSCs

Mesenchymal stem/stromal cells (MSCs) are cell populations with unique hematopoietic-supporting and immunoregulatory properties, which are currently recognized as the uppermost counterparts for regenerative medicine in the field [14]. Since the first isolation from bone marrow, MSCs with various origins have been identified including adult tissues and perinatal tissues such as adipose-tissue-derived MSCs (AD-MSCs), dental-pulp-derived MSCs (DPSCs) [15], fetal-liver-derived MSCs (FL-MSCs), amniotic-membrane-derived MSCs (AMSCs), amniotic-fluid-derived MSCs (AF-MSCs), umbilical-cord-derived MSCs (UC-MSCs) [16, 17], placenta-derived MSCs (P-MSCs) [18], supernumerary teeth-derived apical papillary stem cells (SCAP-Ss) [15]. Meanwhile, current progress also highlighted the large-scale generation of MSCs from human pluripotent stem cells (hPSCs) including human embryonic stem cells (hESCs) and human induced PSCs (hiPSCs) as well [19–21].

2.1 Biofunctions of MSCs

As mentioned above, MSCs are heterogeneous populations with advantaged properties, which thus have been largely recognized as the dominating stromal cells in the hematopoietic microenvironment and the splendid "seed" cells for cellular therapy [22]. Not until the year of 2006, the International Society for Cellular Therapy (ISCT) released minimal guidelines for MSC definition including the fibroblast-like plastic-adherent cells, high percentage of subsets with mesenchymal-associated biomarker expression (CD73, CD90, CD105), whereas minimal expression of hematopoietic-associated (CD31, CD34) or immune-related (HLA-DR) surface markers and multi-lineage differentiation potential toward adipocytes, osteoblasts, and chondrocytes [23]. Of the biofunctions, immunomodulation is of great importance for the translational purposes of MSCs and the derivatives in tissue engineering and regenerative medicine via simultaneously inhibiting and stimulating the immune system and secreting immunosuppressors [24].

To date, MSCs have been extensively explored in multiple intractable and recurrent diseases such as acute-on-chronic liver failure (ACLF) [25], acute myocardial infarction (AMI) [26], acute myelogenous leukemia (AML) [27], refractory wounds [28], atopic dermatitis (AD), Crohn's disease (CD) [18], graft-versus-host disease (GvHD) [16], coronavirus disease 2019 (COVID-19)-associated acute lung injury and acute respiratory distress syndrome (ALI/ARDS) [29, 30].

2.2 Regulatory mechanisms of MSCs

Generally, MSCs function mainly via serving as constructive microenvironment for hematogenesis, secretion (autocrine, paracrine), immunomodulation, and differentiation [31–34]. For instance, the orchestration of multiple pathways (e.g., TGF-β, PPAR-γ2, and the Smad3-SOX9-CREB/p300 axis) in MSCs is critical for in vitro differentiation toward the mesodermal lineages [35, 36]. Instead, López-García and Castro-Manrreza verified the TNF-α and IFN-γ in mediating the immunoregulatory capacity of MSCs in the modulation of the immune response [37]. Interestingly, Montesinos and colleagues verified the regulatory effect of TNF-α and IFN-γ for the enhanced expression of ICAM-1 and microvesicle release of BM-MSCs when exposed to an inflammatory environment [38]. As to bone-marrow-derived MSCs (BM-MSCs), Zhang et al. demonstrated the hyperactivation of JAK–STAT signaling in AML patients compared with those in healthy donors [27].

3. MSCs for allergic disease management

As an intractable autoimmune disease with complex pathogenesis, allergic diseases have caused heavy economic and psychological burden to the patients and their families, and in particular, those with relapse and resistance against drugs. For the purpose, autogenous and allogeneic MSCs with unique bidirectional immunomodulatory property have caught the attention of pioneering investigators in the field. To date, MSCs have been involved in various subtypes of allergic disease management with considerable efficacy such as allergic rhinitis, allergic dermatitis, allergic asthma, and urticaria.

3.1 MSCs for allergic rhinitis management

Allergic rhinitis (AR), a well-described disease entity with extra-nasal manifestations, is considered as a major and increasing chronic inflammatory disease in the respiratory tract [39–41]. The pathogenesis of AR is associated with inflammatory mediators (e.g., IgE) and sensitized mast cells in the submucosa of the upper aerodigestive tract, which is also involved in various upper airway diseases including otitis media, chronic laryngitis, oral allergy syndrome, and obstructive sleep apnea [40, 42–44]. Clinically, although with certain disadvantages such as repeated attacks and adverse reaction, a series of desensitizing drugs including nasal glucocorticoids and antihistamines, together with acupuncture, are currently in use for allergic rhinitis treatment [39, 45–47].

Recently, Zheng et al. investigated the outcomes of 70 patients with allergic rhinitis with the administration of azelastine hydrochloride and montelukast sodium and found that clinical symptom score (e.g., nasal itching, runny nose, and nasal congestion) and serum levels of proinflammatory factors (e.g., hsCRP, IL-6, and IL-8) revealed preferable improvement compared with those 67 patients with azelastine hydrochloride alone [48]. Simultaneously, Xiong et al. recently reported the ameliorative effect of Chinese herbs (e.g., Guominjian) upon AR by utilizing the anti-inflammatory, anti-allergic, and immunomodulatory effects [49]. However, the spectrum of AR and the complex immunopathology further affect the efficacy of antiallergic drugs including antihistamines and mast cell stabilizers and thus, limit the treatment with the concomitant corticosteroid. Moreover, the recurrence of AR has been considered difficult to handle by current drug therapy.

Of note, pioneering clinicians have turned to MSC-based remedy for further improvement in the management of AR based on the immunomodulatory properties. For example, two interventional studies (NCT05167552, NCT05151133) have been registered according to the Clinicaltrials.gov website, and a total number of 78 participants are being enrolled for further treatment with various doses (low dose, 0.5×10^6 cells/kg; moderate dose, 1.0×10^6 cells/kg; high dose, 2.0×10^6 cells/kg) of hUC-MSC infusion (**Table 1**).

3.2 MSCs for atopic dermatitis management

Atopic dermatitis (AD), also regarded as atopic eczema, is a relapsing inflammatory skin condition and a chronic heterogeneous skin lesion worldwide among childhood, infancy, and even adulthood, and in particular, among those families with a history of allergic diseases [50–52]. To date, a variety of pathogenic factors associated with the environmental, immunologic, and genetic elements have been identified for the intrinsic and extrinsic subtypes of AD such as food allergies, respiratory diseases, autoimmune disorders, and inflammatory skin infections [50, 53]. For example, the well-established ingredients including dysbiosis of skin microbiota, epidermal barrier disruption, overactivation of the helper T cell subsets (e.g., Th1, Th2, Th17, Th22), together with increased immunoglobulin E (IgE) and eosinophils in blood, have been demonstrated in association with the pathogenesis of AD [54, 55]. Of the disease progression, the impaired skin barrier is considered as the initial step during the development of AD, which is adequate to cause further allergic sensitization and skin inflammation [56]. Simultaneously, AD is deemed to the initiation phase of relevant atopic disorders such as food allergy and allergic asthma and rhinitis, which is continuous for ages and maintains the relapsing-remitting status in numerous patients [57].

Therewith, despite the current pharmacological and nonpharmacological treatment modalities in relieving misery in patients with moderate to severe AD, the efficacy or persistence is still unsatisfactory on account of the indeterminacy and complexity of the underlying pathogenesis [1, 52]. Strikingly, Kim et al. reported the safety and certain improvements of AD inpatients with an overall response rate of 55% at week 12 with a high dose of hUC-MSC (5×10^7) administration through local subcutaneous injection [58]. Similarly, our group further reported the real cure of an elderly patient rather than partial remission by conducting a single round of

Conditions	NCT no.	Status	Phases	Enroll	Location
Allergic rhinitis	NCT05167552	Not yet recruiting	P1, P2	60	—
	NCT05151133	Recruiting	P1	18	China
Allergic dermatitis	NCT02888704	Completed	P1	13	Korea
	NCT03252340	Active, not recruiting		11	Korea
	NCT04179760	Recruiting	P1, P2	92	Korea
	NCT04137562	Recruiting	P2	118	Korea
Urticaria	NCT02824393	Completed	Early P1	10	Turkey

Table 1.
MSC-based clinical trials upon atopic diseases.

intravenous injection of hUC-MSCs without recrudesce during the 14-month's follow-up. Overall, the aforementioned proof-of-concept studies ulteriorly highlighted the feasibility upon AD patients with refractory AD-associated symptoms.

3.3 MSCs for allergic asthma management

Allergic asthma, known as a "syndrome" with over 300 million individuals worldwide, which also has become a dominating burden in Westernized societies [59].

Generally, allergic asthma is caused by a complex interplay between environmental stimulus and genetic and factors [60, 61]. As a chronic airway inflammatory disease, patients with allergic asthma reveal multifaceted clinical manifestations such as intermittent attacks of airway hyper-reactivity, breathlessness, coughing, and wheezing. As to adult asthma, an initial exposure to allergen triggers Th2 cell-dependent immune response that regulates the production of IgE and cytokines in the lungs [60]. Distinguishing from the characteristics of ILC2s in chronic allergic diseases, IgE sensitization has been considered acting as a crucial role in the progression of allergic diseases [60, 62, 63]. Collectively, the environmental and genetic factors orchestrate the complexity and challenges of allergic asthma posed for the further development of novel remedies for effective treatment and prevention of allergic asthma.

State-of-the-art updates have suggested the therapeutic effect of MSCs or MSC-derived exosomes (MSC-Exo) in the management of allergic asthma in preclinical and clinical investigations [64–66]. For instance, Boldrini-Leite et al. took advantage of the ovalbumin-induced allergic asthma mice model for the remodeling of the inflammatory process and pulmonary symptoms and confirmed the potential of BM-MSCs to modulate lung inflammatory processes and tissue repair. Recently, Huang et al. found that the mitochondrial dysfunction and asthma pathophysiology in the asthma animal model were efficiently rescued by MSC injection, and the levels of relevant gene expression were reversed as well such as interleukins (e.g., IL-4, IL-5, IL-13, IL-25, IL-33) and mitochondria genes (e.g., COX-1, COX-2, Cytb, ND-1) and inflammatory factors (e.g., INF-γ) [65]. Similarly, de Castro et al. demonstrated the efficacy of human adipose tissue–derived MSCs (hAD-MSCs) and the extracellular vesicles upon experimental allergic asthma by airway remodeling. In detail, C57BL/6 female mice with experimental allergic asthma manifested reduced eosinophils in lung tissue, collagen fiber content in lung parenchyma and airways, levels of Tgf-β in lung tissue, and $CD3^{+}CD4^{+}$ T lymphocyte counts in the thymus [67]. Interestingly, Abreu and colleagues verified the enhanced therapeutic effect of MSCs upon allergic asthma by pretreatment with eicosapentaenoic acid (EPA) [68]. Moreover, serum from asthmatic mice has been proved with potentiated efficacy of MSCs in experimental allergic asthma [69]. Taken together, MSCs of different origins alone or in combination with relevant remedies reveal rosy prospective in allergic asthma management.

3.4 MSCs for urticaria management

Urticaria, including the immunological and nonimmunological subtypes, is a series of common skin disorder occurring in 0.5–5% of the general population that affects individuals of all ages and results from many different stimuli, which compromise quality of life and affect individual performance physically and mentally [70–73]. Generally, urticaria acts as a hypersensitivity reaction with mast cell activation due to the stimulation of T lymphocytes and/or antibodies. Instead, nonimmunological urticarias with mast cell activation are involved in immunomodulation (e.g., Toll-like, complement, proinflammatory factors) or toxicity of xenobiotics (e.g., haptens, drugs). Therewith, the variations in the pathophysiological mechanisms further result in the great heterogeneity of clinical symptoms and the variable remedies [72, 74].

Urticaria exhibits multifaceted clinical manifestations such as intensely pruritic wheals, edema of the interstitial or subcutaneous tissue. In details, distinguishing from the acute urticaria, chronic urticaria, including chronic spontaneous urticaria (CSU) and chronic inducible urticaria (e.g., cold urticaria), is regarded as a difficult-to-treat skin disease and results in the major impact on quality of life in patients according to the European guideline on the management of urticaria, which describes a multidisciplinary approach for urticaria administration [75–77].

Being obscure in fully elucidating the underlying etiopathogenesis as well as the limitation in urticaria management, pioneering scientists and clinicians turned to MSC-based cytotherapy for developing more efficient treatment options [73]. Of note, Özgül Özdemir and colleagues employed autologous AD-MSCs for the administration of 10 refractory CSU patients and noticed the immunomodulatory effect upon $CD4^{+}$ T cell subsets and cytokine expression profiling. For instance, the Th2 subset and pro-inflammatory factors (e.g., TGF-β1, IDO, PGE2, anti-FcεRI) revealed a significant decrease in urticaria patients with MSC injection after 2 weeks [73]. Collectively, despite the minimal literatures in the field, the findings suggested that MSCs might be an alternative and effective strategy for treatment-resistant CSU patients in clinical practice [73].

4. Clinical trials of MSC-based remedy for allergic diseases

In the recent years, MSC-based cytotherapy has attracted the attention of a certain number of biologists and clinicians in the field for allergic disease management. According to the Clinicaltrials.gov website of National Institutes of Health (NIH), a total number of seven clinical trials have been registered worldwide (up to May 24th, 2022) including four trials in Korea (NCT02888704, NCT03252340, NCT04179760, NCT04137562), one trial in China (NCT05151133), one trial in Turkey (NCT02824393), and one trial unknowable (NCT05167552) (**Table 1**).

The interventional studies conducted by clinical investigators are designed to explore the safety and effectiveness of MSC-based treatment for relevant disease treatment including two trials for allergic rhinitis, four trials for allergic dermatitis, and one trial for urticaria (**Table 1**). Of the aforementioned clinical trials, two were not yet recruiting, three were recruiting, four were completed, and two were completed (**Table 1**). Meanwhile, we further noticed that all of the registered clinical trials were in the Phase 1 and Phase 2 stages (**Table 1**).

5. Conclusions

MSCs and the concomitant derivatives have emerged as advantaged and alternative sources for allergic disease management. MSC- or MSC-exo/small secretory vesicles (sEVs)-based cytotherapy has supplied overwhelming new tissue engineering platforms to sequentially ameliorate disease manifestations and improve the clinical outcomes of patients with relevant allergic diseases. However, the lack of standardized methodology and evaluation criteria (e.g., safety, effectiveness, biodistribution) in the preparation of good manufacturing practices (GMP)-grade MSCs for clinical purposes hinders the development of MSC-based tissue engineering and regenerative medicine. Therefore, further understanding of the aforementioned aspects of MSCs will benefit clinical applications and the industrialization of MSC-based cytotherapy in future.

Acknowledgements

The authors would like to thank the members in Key Laboratory of Molecular Diagnostics and Precision Medicine for Surgical Oncology in Gansu Province & NHC Key Laboratory of Diagnosis and Therapy of Gastrointestinal Tumor, Gansu Provincial Hospital, and Institute of Biology & Hefei Institute of Physical Science, Chinese Academy of Sciences for their kind suggestions. This study was supported by grants from Science and technology projects of Guizhou Province (QKH-J-ZK[2021]-107), Natural Science Foundation of Jiangxi Province (20212BAB216073), the project Youth Fund funded by Shandong Provincial Natural Science Foundation (ZR2020QC097), the Non-profit Central Research Institute Fund of Chinese Academy of Medical Sciences (2019PT320005), The 2021 Central-Guided Local Science and Technology Development Fund (ZYYDDFFZZJ-1), Gansu Key Laboratory of molecular diagnosis and precision treatment of surgical tumors (18JR2RA033), Key project funded by Department of Science and Technology of Shangrao City (2020AB002, 2020 K003, 2021F013), Jiangxi Provincial Key New Product Incubation Program Funded by Technical Innovation Guidance Program of Shangrao (2020G002), Natural Science Foundation of Gansu Province (21JR11RA186, 20JR10RA415), Key talent project of Gansu Province of the Organization Department of Gansu provincial Party committee (2020RCXM076), Fujian Provincial Ministerial Finance Special Project (2021XH018).

Conflict of interest

The authors declare no conflict of interest.

Notes/thanks/other declarations

Not applicable.

Appendices and nomenclature

MSCs	mesenchymal stem/stromal cells
EAACI	the European Academy of Allergy and Clinical Immunology
AIT	allergen immunotherapy
AR	allergic rhinitis
AD	atopic dermatitis
IgE	immunoglobulin E
hAD-MSCs	human adipose tissue–derived MSCs
EPA	eicosapentaenoic acid

CSU	chronic spontaneous urticaria
UC-MSCs	Umbilical-cord-derived MSCs
P-MSCs	placenta-derived MSCs
AD-MSCs	adipose-tissue-derived MSCs
DPSCs	dental-pulp-derived MSCs
FL-MSCs	fetal-liver-derived MSCs
AMSCs	amniotic-membrane-derived MSCs
AF-MSCs	amniotic-fluid-derived MSCs
UC-MSCs	umbilical-cord-derived MSCs
P-MSCs	placenta-derived MSCs
hPSCs	human pluripotent stem cells
SCAP-Ss	supernumerary teeth-derived apical papillary stem cells
ISCT	the International Society for Cellular Therapy
hESCs	human embryonic stem cells
hiPSCs	human induced PSCs
MSC-exo	MSC-derived exosomes
sEVs	small secretory vesicles
GMP	good manufacturing practices
AML	acute myelogenous leukemia
CD	Crohn's disease
GvHD	graft-versus-host disease
COVID-19	coronavirus disease 2019
ALI	acute lung injury
ARDS	acute respiratory distress syndrome
AMI	acute myocardial infarction
ACLF	acute-on-chronic liver failure

Author details

Leisheng Zhang[1,2,3,4,5]*, Zhongchao Han[4,5] and Xiaowei Gao[6]*

1 Key Laboratory of Molecular Diagnostics and Precision Medicine for Surgical Oncology in Gansu Province and NHC Key Laboratory of Diagnosis and Therapy of Gastrointestinal Tumor, Gansu Provincial Hospital, Lanzhou, China

2 CAS Key Laboratory of Radiation Technology and Biophysics in Institute of Biology and Hefei Institute of Physical Science, Chinese Academy of Sciences, Hefei, China

3 Center for Cellular Therapies, The First Affiliated Hospital of Shandong First Medical University, Ji-nan, China

4 Jiangxi Research Center of Stem Cell Engineering, Jiangxi Health-Biotech Stem Cell Technology Co. Ltd., Shangrao, China

5 Institute of Health-Biotech, Health-Biotech (Tianjin) Stem Cell Research Institute Co. Ltd, Tianjin, China

6 Department of Otorhinolaryngology, Second Hospital of Tianjin Medical University, Tianjin, China

*Address all correspondence to: leisheng_zhang@163.com and beny51@126.com

References

[1] DeVries A, Vercelli D. Epigenetics in allergic diseases. Current Opinion in Pediatrics. 2015;**27**(6):719-723

[2] Huang Y, Wang G, Wang C. Dietary intervention for allergic disease. Current Pharmaceutical Design. 2014;**20**(6):988-995

[3] Nakao A. Circadian regulation of the biology of allergic disease: Clock disruption can promote allergy. Frontiers in Immunology. 2020;**11**:1237

[4] Rottem M, Gershwin ME, Shoenfeld Y. Allergic disease and autoimmune effectors pathways. Developmental Immunology. 2002;**9**(3):161-167

[5] Agache I, Cojanu C, Laculiceanu A, Rogozea L. Genetics and epigenetics of allergy. Current Opinion in Allergy and Clinical Immunology. 2020;**20**(3):223-232

[6] Costela-Ruiz VJ, Illescas-Montes R, Pavon-Martinez R, Ruiz C, Melguizo-Rodriguez L. Role of mast cells in autoimmunity. Life Sciences. 2018;**209**:52-56

[7] Robbie-Ryan M, Brown M. The role of mast cells in allergy and autoimmunity. Current Opinion in Immunology. 2002;**14**(6):728-733

[8] Dhami S, Nurmatov U, Halken S, Calderon MA, Muraro A, Roberts G, et al. Allergen immunotherapy for the prevention of allergic disease: Protocol for a systematic review. Pediatric Allergy and Immunology. 2016;**27**(3):236-241

[9] Howell MD, Fitzsimons C, Smith PA. JAK/STAT inhibitors and other small molecule cytokine antagonists for the treatment of allergic disease. Annals of Allergy, Asthma & Immunology. 2018;**120**(4):367-375

[10] Tang ML, Lahtinen SJ, Boyle RJ. Probiotics and prebiotics: Clinical effects in allergic disease. Current Opinion in Pediatrics. 2010;**22**(5):626-634

[11] Kukkonen K, Savilahti E, Haahtela T, Juntunen-Backman K, Korpela R, Poussa T, et al. Probiotics and prebiotic galacto-oligosaccharides in the prevention of allergic diseases: A randomized, double-blind, placebo-controlled trial. The Journal of Allergy and Clinical Immunology. 2007;**119**(1):192-198

[12] Lopez-Santamarina A, Gonzalez EG, Lamas A, Mondragon ADC, Regal P, Miranda JM. Probiotics as a possible strategy for the prevention and treatment of allergies. A narrative review. Foods. 2021;**10**(4):701

[13] Ismail IH, Licciardi PV, Tang ML. Probiotic effects in allergic disease. Journal of Paediatrics and Child Health. 2013;**49**(9):709-715

[14] Kulus M, Sibiak R, Stefańska K, Zdun M, Wieczorkiewicz M, Piotrowska-Kempisty H, et al. Mesenchymal stem/stromal cells derived from human and animal perinatal tissues-origins, characteristics, signaling pathways, and clinical trials. Cells. 2021;**10**(12):3278

[15] Yao J, Chen N, Wang X, Zhang L, Huo J, Chi Y, et al. Human supernumerary teeth-derived apical papillary stem cells possess preferable characteristics and efficacy on hepatic fibrosis in mice. Stem Cells International. 2020;**2020**:6489396

[16] Zhao Q, Zhang L, Wei Y, Yu H, Zou L, Huo J, et al. Systematic comparison of hUC-MSCs at various passages reveals the variations of signatures and therapeutic effect on acute graft-versus-host disease. Stem Cell Research & Therapy. 2019;**10**(1):354

[17] Zhang Y, Li Y, Li W, Cai J, Yue M, Jiang L, et al. Therapeutic effect of human umbilical cord mesenchymal stem cells at various passages on acute liver failure in rats. Stem Cells International. 2018;**2018**:7159465

[18] Hou H, Zhang L, Duan L, Liu Y, Han Z, Li Z, et al. Spatio-temporal metabolokinetics and efficacy of human placenta-derived mesenchymal stem/stromal cells on mice with refractory Crohn's-like Enterocutaneous Fistula. Stem Cell Reviews and Reports. 2020;**16**(6):1292-1304

[19] Zhang L, Wei Y, Chi Y, Liu D, Yang S, Han Z, et al. Two-step generation of mesenchymal stem/stromal cells from human pluripotent stem cells with reinforced efficacy upon osteoarthritis rabbits by HA hydrogel. Cell & Bioscience. 2021;**11**(1):6

[20] Wei Y, Hou H, Zhang L, Zhao N, Li C, Huo J, et al. JNKi- and DAC-programmed mesenchymal stem/stromal cells from hESCs facilitate hematopoiesis and alleviate hind limb ischemia. Stem Cell Research & Therapy. 2019;**10**(1):186

[21] Zhang L, Wang H, Liu C, Wu Q, Su P, Wu D, et al. MSX2 initiates and accelerates mesenchymal stem/stromal cell specification of hPSCs by regulating TWIST1 and PRAME. Stem Cell Reports. 2018;**11**(2):497-513

[22] Barilani M, Banfi F, Sironi S, Ragni E, Guillaumin S, Polveraccio F, et al. Low-affinity nerve growth factor receptor (CD271) heterogeneous expression in adult and fetal mesenchymal stromal cells. Scientific Reports. 2018;**8**(1):9321

[23] Horwitz EM, Le Blanc K, Dominici M, Mueller I, Slaper-Cortenbach I, Marini FC, et al. International Society for Cellular T: Clarification of the nomenclature for MSC: The International Society for Cellular Therapy position statement. Cytotherapy. 2005;7(5):393-395

[24] Jiang W, Xu J. Immune modulation by mesenchymal stem cells. Cell Proliferation. 2020;**53**(1):e12712

[25] Lin BL, Chen JF, Qiu WH, Wang KW, Xie DY, Chen XY, et al. Allogeneic bone marrow-derived mesenchymal stromal cells for hepatitis B virus-related acute-on-chronic liver failure: A randomized controlled trial. Hepatology. 2017;**66**(1):209-219

[26] Lim M, Wang W, Liang L, Han ZB, Li Z, Geng J, et al. Intravenous injection of allogeneic umbilical cord-derived multipotent mesenchymal stromal cells reduces the infarct area and ameliorates cardiac function in a porcine model of acute myocardial infarction. Stem Cell Research & Therapy. 2018;**9**(1):129

[27] Zhang L, Chi Y, Wei Y, Zhang W, Wang F, Zhang L, et al. Bone marrow-derived mesenchymal stem/stromal cells in patients with acute myeloid leukemia reveal transcriptome alterations and deficiency in cellular vitality. Stem Cell Research & Therapy. 2021;**12**(1):365

[28] Hocking AM. Mesenchymal stem cell therapy for cutaneous wounds. Advanced Wound Care (New Rochelle). 2012;**1**(4):166-171

[29] Zhang LS, Yu Y, Yu H, Han ZC. Therapeutic prospects of mesenchymal stem/stromal cells in COVID-19

associated pulmonary diseases: From bench to bedside. World Journal of Stem Cells. 2021;**13**(8):1058-1071

[30] Aitong W, Leisheng Z, Hao Y. Visualized analyses of investigations upon mesenchymal stem/stromal cell-based cytotherapy and underlying mechanisms for COVID-19 associated ARDS. Current Stem Cell Research & Therapy. 2022;**17**(1):2-12

[31] Wang X, Lazorchak AS, Song L, Li E, Zhang Z, Jiang B, et al. Immune modulatory mesenchymal stem cells derived from human embryonic stem cells through a trophoblast-like stage. Stem Cells. 2016;**34**(2):380-391

[32] Wei Y, Zhang L, Chi Y, Ren X, Gao Y, Song B, et al. High-efficient generation of VCAM-1(+) mesenchymal stem cells with multidimensional superiorities in signatures and efficacy on aplastic anaemia mice. Cell Proliferation. 2020;**53**(8):e12862

[33] Wu Y, Wang Z, Cao Y, Xu L, Li X, Liu P, et al. Cotransplantation of haploidentical hematopoietic and umbilical cord mesenchymal stem cells with a myeloablative regimen for refractory/relapsed hematologic malignancy. Annals of Hematology. 2013;**92**(12):1675-1684

[34] Zhao M, Liu S, Wang C, Wang Y, Wan M, Liu F, et al. Mesenchymal stem cell-derived extracellular vesicles attenuate mitochondrial damage and inflammation by stabilizing mitochondrial DNA. ACS Nano. 2021;**15**(1):1519-1538

[35] Tontonoz P, Hu E, Spiegelman BM. Stimulation of adipogenesis in fibroblasts by PPAR gamma 2, a lipid-activated transcription factor. Cell. 1994;**79**(7):1147-1156

[36] Furumatsu T, Tsuda M, Taniguchi N, Tajima Y, Asahara H. Smad3 induces chondrogenesis through the activation of SOX9 via CREB-binding protein/p300 recruitment. The Journal of Biological Chemistry. 2005;**280**(9):8343-8350

[37] Lopez-Garcia L, Castro-Manrreza ME. TNF-alpha and IFN-gamma participate in improving the immunoregulatory capacity of mesenchymal stem/stromal cells: Importance of cell-cell contact and extracellular vesicles. International Journal of Molecular Sciences. 2021;**22**(17)

[38] Montesinos JJ, Lopez-Garcia L, Cortes-Morales VA, Arriaga-Pizano L, Valle-Rios R, Fajardo-Orduna GR, et al. Human bone marrow mesenchymal stem/stromal cells exposed to an inflammatory environment increase the expression of ICAM-1 and release microvesicles enriched in this adhesive molecule: Analysis of the Participation of TNF-alpha and IFN-gamma. Journal of Immunology Research. 2020;**2020**:8839625

[39] Bao H, Si D, Gao L, Sun H, Shi Q, Yan Y, et al. Acupuncture for the treatment of allergic rhinitis: A systematic review protocol. Medicine (Baltimore). 2018;**97**(51):e13772

[40] Mur T, Brook C, Platt M. Extranasal manifestations of allergy in the head and neck. Current Allergy and Asthma Reports. 2020;**20**(7):21

[41] Cassano M, Maselli A, Mora F, Cassano P. Rhinobronchial syndrome: Pathogenesis and correlation with allergic rhinitis in children. International Journal of Pediatric Otorhinolaryngology. 2008;**72**(7):1053-1058

[42] Martines F, Salvago P, Ferrara S, Messina G, Mucia M, Plescia F, et al. Factors influencing the development of otitis media among Sicilian children

affected by upper respiratory tract infections. Brazilian Journal of Otorhinolaryngology. 2016;**82**(2):215-222

[43] Fireman P. Otitis media and eustachian tube dysfunction: Connection to allergic rhinitis. The Journal of Allergy and Clinical Immunology. 1997;**99**(2):S787-S797

[44] Ciprandi G, Tosca MA. Turbinate hypertrophy, allergic rhinitis, and otitis media. Current Allergy and Asthma Reports. 2021;**21**(9):44

[45] Li J, Liu L, Jiao L, Liao K, Xu L, Zhou X, et al. Clinical acupuncture therapy for children with allergic rhinitis: A protocol for systematic review and meta analysis. Medicine (Baltimore). 2021;**100**(3):e24086

[46] Feng S, Han M, Fan Y, Yang G, Liao Z, Liao W, et al. Acupuncture for the treatment of allergic rhinitis: A systematic review and meta-analysis. American Journal of Rhinology & Allergy. 2015;**29**(1):57-62

[47] Bai H, Xu S, Wu Q, Xu S, Sun K, Wu J, et al. Clinical events associated with acupuncture intervention for the treatment of chronic inflammation associated disorders. Mediators of Inflammation. 2020;**2020**:2675785

[48] Zheng Q, Ma D, Zhu Q, Tang S, Chen C. Effect of azelastine hydrochloride combined with montelukast sodium in the treatment of patients with allergic rhinitis. American Journal of Translational Research. 2021;**13**(8):9570-9577

[49] Xiong Y, Li H, Zhang SN. Guominjian for allergic rhinitis: A protocol for systematic review and meta-analysis of randomized clinical trials. Medicine (Baltimore). 2020;**99**(44):e22854

[50] Torres T, Ferreira EO, Goncalo M, Mendes-Bastos P, Selores M, Filipe P. Update on atopic dermatitis. Acta Médica Portuguesa. 2019;**32**(9):606-613

[51] Cabanillas B, Brehler AC, Novak N. Atopic dermatitis phenotypes and the need for personalized medicine. Current Opinion in Allergy and Clinical Immunology. 2017;**17**(4):309-315

[52] Stander S. Atopic dermatitis. The New England Journal of Medicine. 2021;**384**(12):1136-1143

[53] Leung DY, Nicklas RA, Li JT, Bernstein IL, Blessing-Moore J, Boguniewicz M, et al. Disease management of atopic dermatitis: An updated practice parameter. Joint Task Force on Practice Parameters. Annals of Allergy, Asthma & Immunology. 2004;**93**(3 Suppl 2):S1-S21

[54] Guttman-Yassky E, Nograles KE, Krueger JG. Contrasting pathogenesis of atopic dermatitis and psoriasis—Part II: Immune cell subsets and therapeutic concepts. The Journal of Allergy and Clinical Immunology. 2011;**127**(6):1420-1432

[55] Suarez-Farinas M, Dhingra N, Gittler J, Shemer A, Cardinale I, de Guzman SC, et al. Intrinsic atopic dermatitis shows similar TH2 and higher TH17 immune activation compared with extrinsic atopic dermatitis. The Journal of Allergy and Clinical Immunology. 2013;**132**(2):361-370

[56] Kim J, Kim BE, Leung DYM. Pathophysiology of atopic dermatitis: Clinical implications. Allergy and Asthma Proceedings. 2019;**40**(2):84-92

[57] Schneider L, Tilles S, Lio P, Boguniewicz M, Beck L, LeBovidge J, et al. Atopic dermatitis: A practice parameter update 2012. The Journal

of Allergy and Clinical Immunology. 2013;**131**(2):295-299

[58] Kim HS, Yun JW, Shin TH, Lee SH, Lee BC, Yu KR, et al. Human umbilical cord blood mesenchymal stem cell-derived PGE2 and TGF-beta1 alleviate atopic dermatitis by reducing mast cell degranulation. Stem Cells. 2015;**33**(4):1254-1266

[59] Eigenmann PA. Diagnosis of allergy syndromes: Do symptoms always mean allergy? Allergy. 2005;**60**(Suppl 79):6-9

[60] Mukherjee AB, Zhang Z. Allergic asthma: Influence of genetic and environmental factors. The Journal of Biological Chemistry. 2011;**286**(38):32883-32889

[61] Gaber T, Chen Y, Krauss PL, Buttgereit F. Metabolism of T lymphocytes in health and disease. International Review of Cell and Molecular Biology. 2019;**342**:95-148

[62] Leffler J, Stumbles PA, Strickland DH. Immunological processes driving IgE sensitisation and disease development in males and females. International Journal of Molecular Sciences. 2018;**19**(6)

[63] Doherty TA. At the bench: Understanding group 2 innate lymphoid cells in disease. Journal of Leukocyte Biology. 2015;**97**(3):455-467

[64] Ren J, Liu Y, Yao Y, Feng L, Zhao X, Li Z, et al. Intranasal delivery of MSC-derived exosomes attenuates allergic asthma via expanding IL-10 producing lung interstitial macrophages in mice. International Immunopharmacology. 2021;**91**:107288

[65] Huang M, Mehrabi Nasab E, Athari SS. Immunoregulatory effect of mesenchymal stem cell via mitochondria signaling pathways in allergic asthma. Saudi Journal of Biological Science. 2021;**28**(12):6957-6962

[66] Abreu SC, Antunes MA, de Castro JC, de Oliveira MV, Bandeira E, Ornellas DS, et al. Bone marrow-derived mononuclear cells vs. mesenchymal stromal cells in experimental allergic asthma. Respiratory Physiology & Neurobiology. 2013;**187**(2):190-198

[67] de Castro LL, Xisto DG, Kitoko JZ, Cruz FF, Olsen PC, Redondo PAG, et al. Human adipose tissue mesenchymal stromal cells and their extracellular vesicles act differentially on lung mechanics and inflammation in experimental allergic asthma. Stem Cell Research & Therapy. 2017;**8**(1):151

[68] Abreu SC, Lopes-Pacheco M, da Silva AL, Xisto DG, de Oliveira TB, Kitoko JZ, et al. Eicosapentaenoic acid enhances the effects of mesenchymal stromal cell therapy in experimental allergic asthma. Frontiers in Immunology. 2018;**9**:1147

[69] Abreu SC, Xisto DG, de Oliveira TB, Blanco NG, de Castro LL, Kitoko JZ, et al. Serum from asthmatic mice potentiates the therapeutic effects of mesenchymal stromal cells in experimental allergic asthma. Stem Cells Translational Medicine. 2019;**8**(3):301-312

[70] Kulthanan K, Tuchinda P, Chularojanamontri L, Chanyachailert P, Korkij W, Chunharas A, et al. Clinical practice guideline for diagnosis and management of urticaria. Asian Pacific Journal of Allergy and Immunology. 2016;**34**(3):190-200

[71] Monroe EW, Jones HE. Urticaria. An updated review. Archives in Dermatology. 1977;**113**(1):80-90

[72] Hennino A, Berard F, Guillot I, Saad N, Rozieres A, Nicolas JF.

Pathophysiology of urticaria. Clinical Reviews in Allergy and Immunology. 2006;**30**(1):3-11

[73] Ozgul Ozdemir RB, Ozdemir AT, Kirmaz C, Ovali E, Olmez E, Kerem H, et al. Mesenchymal stem cells: A potential treatment approach for refractory chronic spontaneous urticaria. Stem Cell Reviews and Reports. 2021;**17**(3):911-922

[74] Saini SS. Chronic spontaneous urticaria: Etiology and pathogenesis. Immunology and Allergy Clinics of North America. 2014;**34**(1):33-52

[75] Sabroe RA. Acute urticaria. Immunology and Allergy Clinics of North America. 2014;**34**(1):11-21

[76] Alcantara Villar M, Armario Hita JC, Cimbollek S, Fernandez Ballesteros MD, Galan Gutierrez M, Hernandez Montoya C, et al. A review of the latest recommendations on the management of chronic urticaria: A Multidisciplinary Consensus Statement from Andalusia, Spain. Actas Dermosifiliogr (Engl Ed). 2020;**111**(3):222-228

[77] Maltseva N, Borzova E, Fomina D, Bizjak M, Terhorst-Molawi D, Kosnik M, et al. Cold urticaria—What we know and what we do not know. Allergy. 2021;**76**(4):1077-1094

Chapter 8

Perspective Chapter: Management of Allergic Diseases during Pandemic

Öner Özdemir and Emine Aylin Yilmaz

Abstract

Over the recent time period, pediatric allergy clinics across the world have markedly changed their practice because of the COVID-19 pandemic. Nowadays, clinics are not inclined to accept a patient demanding a new procedure / therapeutic modality during pandemic. All allergic diseases require continuous management and treatment, and their socioeconomic burden has been increasing worldwide. In this chapter, the aim is to focus on allergic diseases management during pandemic. During this time, patient follow-up, patient management, and diagnostic tests are real challenges. Limited face-to-face consultations and as much as use of telemedicine are currently seen as the major issues in the allergy practice. Face-to-face examination and treatment should be preferred only in vital situations. During COVID-19 pandemic, patient education, which is the most important step in the treatment of allergic diseases, has started to be done online. The prevailing opinion in the allergy community is that the treatment should not be interrupted, or dose reduction should not be made. According to the guidelines, it is appropriately recommended to carefully calculate the profit and loss of the treatment on a case-by-case basis.

Keywords: allergic diseases, allergy, pandemic, COVID-19, SARS-CoV-2

1. Introduction

Throughout the World, admission to the hospital was restricted during the pandemic, except for emergencies. Over the recent time period, pediatric allergy clinics across the world have markedly changed their practice because of the COVID-19 pandemic. All allergic diseases require continuous management and treatment, and their socioeconomic burden has been increasing worldwide [1]. On top of it, the prevalence of allergic diseases has been dramatically increasing in the world [1]. In this chapter, the aim is to focus on the management of allergic disorders, disease by disease, during pandemic.

2. Allergic rhinitis

Allergic rhinitis is a very common disease that impairs quality of life if left untreated. Although the prevalence of allergic rhinitis is between 10% and 58,5%

worldwide, it varies widely [2]. Allergic rhinitis is an immunoglobulin E (IgE) mediated allergic disease. Allergic patients manifest with symptoms of rhinitis and conjunctivitis, nasal itching, rhinorrhea, nasal congestion, cough, postnasal drip, and sneezing [3]. According to the guidelines, the diagnosis must be confirmed by a skin test and laboratory.

The allergic rhinitis treatment is composed of three major categories: environmental control measures or allergen avoidance, pharmacological treatment, and specific allergen immunotherapy.

Intranasal corticosteroid therapy for these patients can be questionable. But there is no evidence that such therapy can cause immunosuppression. Considering the frequency of hospitalization and mortality in allergic rhinitis patients, it has been observed that these allergic diseases do not pose a risk for COVID-19 [4]. Current therapy cessation is not recommended [3].

3. Anaphylaxis

The lifetime prevalence of anaphylaxis is estimated at 0,05–3% in USA and Europe [5]. Anaphylaxis is a potentially life-threatening, severe allergic reaction. The patient or medical doctor should not refrain from administering epinephrine as soon as they suspect anaphylaxis. During the pandemic, the average number of daily admissions to the emergency department has reported a significant drop. The severity of anaphylaxis symptoms is the main determinant of hospital admission. In particular, the number of food-related anaphylaxis may have decreased as a result of the closure of restaurants. The management of anaphylaxis during the pandemic, the most important point is to be able to immediately administer epinephrine. The use of epinephrine autoinjector as soon as possible is critical in reducing the severity of anaphylaxis symptoms. After that, patients should be monitored for treatment and symptoms (e.g., hypotension, wheezing, shortness of breath, vomiting, and swelling). Although applications to the emergency departments have decreased during the pandemic, it should not be delayed for a patient with anaphylaxis to present or be taken to the emergency department.

4. Asthma

Asthma is a chronic disease usually characterized by chronic reversible obstructive airway inflammation. The fluctuating clinical symptoms are shortness of breath, wheezing, chest tightness, and cough [3].

Asthma prevalence rates vary by country and by age [6]. During pandemic, performing spirometry and reversibility tests have been canceled in the beginning [7]. Later, various organizations formulated operational measures for resuming the functioning of pulmonary function test laboratories [8].

Asthmatic patients have to be managed carefully. T-helper 2 polarization might impair the efficient antiviral immune response [9, 10]. Asthmatic patients also have a greater susceptibility to respiratory viral infections, which may be a trigger for exacerbations [11, 12]. It is critically important to keep the disease under control in asthma patients [13, 14]. Discontinuation of therapy may exacerbate the underlying disease, which may adversely affect the clinic in patients infected with COVID-19.

Many publications recommend that the inhaled steroid dose be maintained at the same dose. However, opinions have been presented that systemic (orally/parenterally administered) corticosteroid therapy could be risky [7].

According to the ARIA-EAACI statement, "If you stop or modify your treatment, you run the risk that your allergic disease, particularly your asthma control, could become worse, causing you to need rescue medications or be admitted to the hospital." [5]. Continuation of anti-IgE (omalizumab) and other biological therapy (mepolizumab, enralizumab, etc.) is recommended during the follow-up of patients with severe asthma [15, 16].

In order to reduce the risk of SARS-CoV-2 transmission, it is preferred to treat the asthma attack at home with metered dose inhaler (MDI), and avoiding nebulizer treatment in the emergency services [7, 17].

When the COVID-19 pandemic emerged, concerns were also raised regarding the safety of allergen immunotherapy. Current studies demonstrated adherence by clinicians to national and international position papers and guidelines of allergen immunotherapy during the COVID-19 pandemic worldwide. Besides, several surveys/research have shown good tolerability of allergen immunotherapy for both subcutaneous and sublingual-oral forms [18].

Fortunately, the hospitalization frequency and time are not significantly increased in asthmatic patients more than in non-asthmatic patients since the pandemic asthma management becomes more complicated.

5. Atopic dermatitis

Atopic dermatitis prevalence is estimated up to 15–20% in the pediatric population and 1–3% in adults worldwide [19]. Focusing on atopic patients, the treatment plan (dosage, drug frequency) is not changed (not recommended to step down medication). It is also known that in patients with atopic dermatitis, the skin barrier is generally disrupted. For this reason, it is recommended to moisturize the skin frequently to avoid exacerbation of complaints.

There is no evidence that patients with barrier defects have a higher risk of SARS-CoV-2 infection or skin complications during COVID-19 [3]. Considering the frequency of hospitalization and mortality in atopic patients, it has been observed that these allergic diseases do not pose a risk for COVID-19. However, classic immunosuppressants or systemic glucocorticoids are not recommended in patients with severe atopic dermatitis due to broad immunosuppressive effects [3, 20, 21].

6. Food allergy

Food allergy can result in a life-threatening anaphylactic reaction. The prevalence of food allergy is generally higher in children than in adults, with a rate of 1–10% [22].

The visits of food-allergic children should be limited to those that are unequivocally needed on a clinical basis. During the pandemic, oral food challenges could be performed in just selected cases [23]. It is recommended to continue the current food diet. In preschool-aged children, accidental food allergic reactions were rarer. Since the food choice is made by the caregiver at preschool-aged, food allergy reaction is less common.

7. Urticaria- Angioedema

Roughly 15–23% of adults have experienced at least one acute urticaria episode at some time in their lifetime, and the prevalence of chronic urticaria in adults is estimated at 0,5–5% [24].

During the pandemic, the approach to urticaria patients differed from other allergic diseases. Because urticaria is one of the most common cutaneous manifestations of COVID-19. These patients were treated with oral antihistamines as well as oral steroids [25]. There was an increase in the frequency of admission to hospital with urticaria. There are many cases of urticaria associated with COVID-19 in the literature [12]. This situation should not be overlooked before the patient is evaluated as urticaria and treatment are started. Further evaluation and possible allergy tests and diagnostic procedures were canceled during pandemic. Only patients who needed hospital treatment that could not be postponed were hospitalized.

Immediate (type I) hypersensitivity reactions develop within 4–6 hours after COVID-19 vaccination and are mediated through Ig E-dependent mediator release. In the case of COVID-19 vaccines, polyethylene glycols and cross-reactive polysorbate 80 have been held responsible to be the triggering factors for immediate reactions. Type I reactions may range from mild, with urticaria-angioedema only, to life-threatening with anaphylaxis [26]. The most common reaction was urticaria followed by various skin rashes, that is, morbilliform, pityriasis rosea-like eruption, bullous drug reactions, fixed drug eruption, etc.

Acute urticaria only after any mRNA or CoronaVac vaccination should not be contraindicated for revaccination. Anaphylaxis to the first dose may be a contraindication to succeeding mRNA vaccination; however, various mild or nonimmediate allergic reactions are not. Type I allergic reactions after dose 1 of mRNA vaccine may contribute to unfinished vaccination. Allergists should be prepared to guide these kinds of subjects to preclude partial vaccination [27, 28].

Patients with urticaria were treated mainly with oral antihistamines. Oral steroids can also be used in therapy. Low-dose systemic steroids with antihistamines have been

Allergic disease type	Treatment/follow-up recommendations
Allergic rhinitis	Intranasal corticosteroid cessation or interruption is not recommended [4, 5].
Anaphylaxis	The most dangerous life-threatening allergic disease is anaphylaxis and epinephrine administration is highly recommended as soon as anaphylaxis is suspected.
Asthma	Medication cessation may lead to asthma exacerbations [5, 13]. It is recommended to continue biologic therapy with anti-IgE or anti-IL-5 in patients with severe asthma [15, 16]. Many publications recommend that the inhaled steroid dose be maintained at the same dose. However, opinions have been presented that systemic (orally/parenterally administered) corticosteroid therapy is could be risky [8].
Atopic dermatitis	It is not recommended to step down medication [20, 21]. Frequent skin moistening is recommended.
Food allergy	It is recommended to continue the current food diet.
Urticaria - Angioedema	Urticarial patients were treated mainly with oral antihistamines. Oral steroids can also be used in therapy [25, 29].

Table 1.
Recently recommendations on allergic diseases.

reported to effectively manage severe urticaria in patients [29]. **Table 1** summarizes the approach to allergic diseases during the COVID-19 pandemic.

8. COVID vaccine side effects in allergic diseases

Due to the "SARS-CoV-2" that started in 2019, there has been a challenging global pandemic process. One of the most effective public health interventions modern medicine has to offer is vaccination. No fatal cases have been reported in vaccine-related allergic reactions. According to a large population-based study, the frequency of vaccine-related allergic reactions is 1.31 (95%CI, 0.90–1.84) cases per million vaccine doses [30]. COVID-19 vaccines can cause a wide range of adverse effects from lymphadenopathy to pain at the injection site [31], but the allergic reaction mechanism, immediate or delayed, is unknown [32]. Side effects such as axillary tenderness, lymphadenopathy, nausea, vomiting, erythema/swelling/pain at the site of injection, fever, joint pain, chills, myalgia, headache, and fatigue are considered as mild reactions [31]. Both vaccines have rarely had serious side effects, including anaphylaxis. According to meta-analysis, the allergic reaction incidence is reported to be higher with the Moderna vaccine [31]. Besides, the excipients that are held responsible for allergic reactions are inactive ingredients that boost the immune response and prevent contamination [30]. Given the importance of the vaccine in fighting this public health crisis, understanding the allergic reactions to the US Food and Drug Administration (FDA) approved vaccines is pivotal [30]. On the other side, the Moderna vaccine has advantages over the Pfizer vaccine in terms of transport and storage [31].

Table 2 summarizes the COVID-19 vaccine's properties and schedule.

	Pfizer/BioNTech vaccine	**Moderna vaccine**
Type	mRNA (BNT162b2)	mRNA (mRNA-1273)
Dose	Each dose contains 30 ug (0.3 mL)	Each dose contains 50 ug (0.5 mL)
Injection number/Period	2 shots, 21 days apart	2 shots, 28 days apart
Age group	6 months of age and older	6 months of age and older
Effectiveness	95% preventative	94.5% preventative
Mechanism of immunity	Into host cells to allow expression of the SARS-CoV-2 S antigen.	Into host cells to allow expression of the SARS-CoV-2 S antigen.

Table 2.
The COVID-19 mRNA vaccination schedule [31].

9. Conclusion

During pandemic, patient management, follow-up, and diagnostic tests are the real challenge. Limited face-to-face consultations and as much as the use of telemedicine is currently seen as the major issues in the allergy practice. Face-to-face examination and treatment should be preferred only in vital situations [33]. The treatment of allergic patients should not be interrupted, or dose reduction should not be made. According to the guidelines, it is recommended to carefully weigh the benefits and losses of the management on a case-by-case basis [34].

Author details

Öner Özdemir[1*] and Emine Aylin Yılmaz[2]

1 Research and Training Hospital of Sakarya University Faculty of Medicine, Division of Allergy and Immunology, Sakarya, Türkiye

2 Research and Training Hospital of Sakarya University Faculty of Medicine, Department of Pediatrics, Sakarya, Türkiye

*Address all correspondence to: ozdemir_oner@hotmail.com

References

[1] Choi HG, Kong IG. Asthma, allergic rhinitis, and atopic dermatitis incidence in Korean adolescents before and after COVID-19. Journal of Clinical Medicine. 2021;**10**(15):3446. DOI: 10.3390/jcm10153446

[2] Kef K, Güven S. The prevalence of allergic rhinitis and associated risk factors among University Students in Anatolia. Journal of Asthma Allergy. 2020;**13**:589-597. DOI: 10.2147/JAA.S279916

[3] Izquierdo-Domínguez A, Rojas-Lechuga MJ, Alobid I. Management of allergic diseases during COVID-19 outbreak. Current Allergy and Asthma Reports. 2021;**21**(2):8. DOI: 10.1007/s11882-021-00989-x

[4] Gani F et al. Allergic rhinitis and COVID-19: Friends or foes? European Annals of Allergy Clinical Immunology. 2022;**54**(2):53-59. DOI: 10.23822/EurAnnACI.1764-1489.234

[5] Bousquet J et al. Intranasal corticosteroids in allergic rhinitis in COVID-19 infected patients: An ARIA-EAACI statement. Allergy: European Journal of Allergy and Clinical Immunology. 2020;**75**(10):2440-2444. DOI: 10.1111/all.14302

[6] S. C. Dharmage, J. L. Perret, and A. Custovic, "Epidemiology of asthma in children and adults," Frontiers in Pediatrics, vol. 7, pp. 1-15, Jun. 2019, DOI: 10.3389/fped.2019.00246

[7] Papadopoulos NG, Custovic A. Impact of COVID-19 on pediatric asthma: Practice adjustments and disease burden. Journal of Allergy and Clinical Immunology: In Practice. 2020;**8**(8):2592-2599.e3. DOI: 10.1016/j.jaip.2020.06.001

[8] Mrigpuri P, Spalgais S, Goel N, Mehta R, Sonal S, Kumar R. A low-cost pulmonary function test laboratory setup for infection control during COVID-19. Lung India. 2022;**39**:93-94. DOI: 10.4103/lungindia.lungindia_578_21

[9] el Shahawy AA, Oladimeji KE, Hamdallah A, Saidani A, Abd-Rabu R, Dahman NBH. Prognosis of COVID-19 in respiratory allergy: a systematic review and meta-analysis. The Egyptian Journal of Biotechnology. 2022;**16**(1):12. DOI: 10.1186/s43168-022-00110-4

[10] Poddighe D, Kovzel E. Impact of anti-type 2 inflammation biologic therapy on COVID-19 clinical course and outcome. Journal of Inflammation Research. 2021;**14**:6845-6853. DOI: 10.2147/JIR.S345665

[11] Liu S, Zhi Y, Ying S. COVID-19 and asthma: Reflection during the pandemic. Clinical Reviews in Allergy and Immunology. 2020;**59**(1):78-88. DOI: 10.1007/s12016-020-08797-3

[12] Özdemir Ö, Nezir Engin MM, Yilmaz EA. COVID-19-related pneumonia in an adolescent patient with allergic asthma. Case Reports in Medicine. 2021;**2021**:1-5. DOI: 10.1155/2021/6706218

[13] Özdemir Ö. Letter to the Editor: Regarding COVID-19 in children with asthma. Lung. 2021;**199**(4):435-436. DOI: 10.1007/s00408-021-00459-1

[14] Özdemir Ö. Asthma and prognosis of coronavirus disease 2019. World Allergy Organization Journal. 2022;**15**(6):100656. DOI: 10.1016/j.waojou.2022.100656

[15] Aksu K et al. COVID-19 in a patient with severe asthma using mepolizumab. Allergy and Asthma Proceedings.

2021;**42**(2):55-57. DOI: 10.2500/AAP.2021.42.200125

[16] Özdemir Ö. Incidence of SARS-CoV-2 infection in asthma patients on omalizumab therapy. Erciyes Medical Journal. 2022;**44**(5):533-534. DOI: 10.14744/etd.2022.28938

[17] Cazzola M, Ora J, Bianco A, Rogliani P, Gabriella M. Since January 2020 Elsevier has created a COVID-19 resource centre with free information in English and Mandarin on the novel coronavirus COVID- 19. The COVID-19 resource centre is hosted on Elsevier Connect, the company' s public news and information. 2020

[18] Pfaar O et al. Allergen immunotherapy during the COVID-19 pandemic—A survey of the German Society for Allergy and Clinical Immunology. Clinical Translational Allergy. 2022;**12**(3):1-8. DOI: 10.1002/clt2.12134

[19] Nutten S. Atopic dermatitis: Global epidemiology and risk factors. Annals of Nutrition and Metabolism. 2015;**66**(Suppl 1):8-16. DOI: 10.1159/000370220

[20] Ricardo JW, Lipner SR. Considerations for safety in the use of systemic medications for psoriasis and atopic dermatitis during the COVID-19 pandemic. Dermatologic Therapy. 2020;**33**(5). DOI: 10.1111/dth.13687

[21] Grieco T et al. Impact of COVID-19 on patients with atopic dermatitis. Clinics in Dermatology. 2021;**39**(6):1083-1087. DOI: 10.1016/j.clindermatol.2021.07.008

[22] Sicherer SH, Sampson HA. Food allergy: A review and update on epidemiology, pathogenesis, diagnosis, prevention, and management. Journal of Allergy and Clinical Immunology. 2017;**141**(1):41-58. DOI: 10.1016/j.jaci.2017.11.003

[23] D'Auria E et al. COVID-19 and food allergy in children. Acta Biomedicine. 2020;**91**(2):204-206. DOI: 10.23750/abm.v91i2.9614

[24] Lee SJ et al. Prevalence and risk factors of urticaria with a focus on chronic urticaria in children. Allergy, Asthma & Immunology Research. 2017;**9**(3):212-219. DOI: 10.4168/aair.2017.9.3.212

[25] Algaadi SA. Urticaria and COVID-19: A review. Dermatologic Therapy. 2020;**33**(6):1-7. DOI: 10.1111/dth.14290

[26] Özdemir Ö. Angioedema following COVID-19 vaccination. Ophthalmic Plastic & Reconstructive Surgery. 2022;**38**(1):97-98. DOI: 10.1097/IOP.0000000000002106

[27] Şeker E, Özdemir Ö. COVID-19 vaccines and hypersensitivity reactions. Chronicles of Precision Medical Researchers. 2022;**3**(1):32-37. DOI: 10.5281/zenodo.6371477

[28] Dikici Ü, Özdemir Ö. Acute urticaria after Pfizer-BioNTech vaccine in adolescent child. Sakarya Medical Journal. 2022;**9561**(2):375-377. DOI: 10.31832/smj.1037264

[29] Şeker E, Pala A, Özdemir Ö. COVID-19 disease and its effect on the follow-up of allergic and immunologic diseases. Sakarya Medical Journal. 2020;**10**(3):514-519. DOI: 10.31832/smj.731345

[30] Banerji A et al. mRNA vaccines to prevent COVID-19 disease and reported allergic reactions: Current evidence and suggested approach. Journal of Allergy and Clinical Immunology: In Practice.

2021;**9**(4):1423-1437. DOI: 10.1016/j.jaip.2020.12.047

[31] Meo SA., Bukhari IA., Akram J., and Klonoff DC. COVID-19 vaccines: Comparison of biological, pharmacological characteristics and adverse effects of Pfizer/BioNTech and Moderna Vaccines. European Review for Medical and Pharmacological Sciences. 2021;**25**(3):1663-1669. DOI: 10.26355/eurrev_202102_24877

[32] Pitlick MM, Joshi AY, Gonzalez-Estrada A, Chiarella SE. Delayed systemic urticarial reactions following mRNA COVID-19 vaccination. Allergy and Asthma Proceedings. 2022;**43**(1):40-43. DOI: 10.2500/aap.2022.43.210101

[33] Edgerley S, Zhu R, Quidwai A, Kim H, Jeimy S. Telemedicine in allergy/immunology in the era of COVID-19: A Canadian perspective. Allergy, Asthma and Clinical Immunology. 2022;**18**(1). DOI: 10.1186/s13223-022-00657-3

[34] Eichenfield LF, Tom WL, Berger TG, Krol A, Paller AS, Schwarzenberger K. Guidelines of care for the management of atopic. Journal of the American Academy of Dermatology. 2015;**71**(1):116-132. DOI: 10.1016/j.jaad.2014.03.023